VITAMINS
MINERAL, SUPPLEMENT &
HERB
DIGEST

Dr. Kumar Pati

New Editions Publishing
30982 Huntwood Avenue, Suite 208
Hayward, California 94544 USA

The material in this book is intended to provide a review of natural therapies. If any treatments described herein are used, they should be undertaken only under the guidance of a licensed health-care practitioner. The authors, editor and publisher assume no responsibility for any adverse outcomes which you derive from your use of any of these treatments in a program of self care or under the care of a licensed practitioner.

Cover Design by **Prabin Badhia**

Library of Congress Catalog Card Number 96-092151 ISBN 0-9624780-7-5

Publishers Cataloging in Publication Data

Pati, Kumar, editor
Vitamin Digest
Includes Index
1. Vitamins
2. Minerals
3. Herbs

PRINTINGS

1st Edition, April 1996
2nd Edition, July 1996
3rd Edition, December, 1996
4th Edition, October, 2002
5th Edition, February, 2003
6th Edition, February, 2004
7th Edition, July 2004
8th Edition, February, 2005

Printed in U.S.A.

DEDICATION

This book is dedicated to all of our friends who have helped us to put together this encyclopedia of vitamins, minerals, herbs and other supplements in digest form.

IN APPRECIATION

- **Dr. Anthony James** *Degidio, D.O. of Ohio for editing & proofreading.*

- **Dr. James Carlson,** *D.C. of Rocklin, california for suggestions.*

- **Monica Valerio** *of Stanford University, California for typing and proofreading.*

- **Don Douglas** *in Germany for compiling all the text and copy editing.*

- **David Loh***, Singapore, Former Regional Executive Director of Macmillan Publishing (Macmillan Southeast Asia) for proofreading.*

- **Richard Tunkel, M.D. and Ann Denis***,for their many helpful suggestions throughout the text*

- **M. A. Vijey,** *AMP., PMC, PJK. Group Managing Director, Big Corp-A Berhad, Kuala Lumpur, Malaysia.*

- **Lina Rueppel,** *of Honolulu, Hawaii for great encauragement.*

- **Meena Sharma,** *M.A. Graphic Designer, New Delhi, India.*

Special Thanks to:-
- **Prabin Badhia***, Emeryville, California, USA for Cover and designing the text.*

- **Felicia Ortega,** *Personal Assistant to Dr. Kumar pati.*

- **Blanquita Antoniadis,** *Melbourne Australia for final proofreading*

FOREWORD

Alternative health, nutritional and herbal therapies are gaining recognition and popularity all over the world. In this digest readers can find information on vitamins, minerals, herbs, supplements drawn from worldwide sources, including Chinese medicine, Indian Ayurveda, and other dietary sciences.

Vitamin Digest is meant to be a guidebook for the general public as well as professionals. Readers with health problems are advised to consult their health care professional.

— Dr. Kumar Pati, Publisher

Contents

VITAMINS

MINERALS

DIETARY SUPPLEMENTS

INDEX
OF
VITAMINS

VITAMIN A

DESCRIPTION

Vitamin A occurs in two forms: preformed vitamin A, known as retinol, and provitamin A, also known as beta carotene. Vitamin A is also known as "the vision vitamin" for its role in aiding eyesight. Because it is fat-soluble and stored in the liver, it need not be replenished every day.

Vitamin A helps maintain healthy skin, teeth and bones, as well as mucous membranes, such as those in the nose, throat and lungs. It is necessary in the formation of an eye pigment involved in night vision, and is therefore essential for vision in dim light. Vitamin A is needed for proper development of the fetus in the womb.

DEFICIENCY SYMPTOMS

Severe deficiency leads to various physical changes in the eye and will eventually lead to blindness. Marginal deficiency will lead to increased susceptibility to respiratory tract infections and skin problems.

THERAPEUTIC USES

- certain skin conditions, e.g. acne and psoriasis

THOSE WHO MAY NEED TO SUPPLEMENT

- vegetarians
- diabetics (who cannot efficiently convert beta carotene into vitamin A)
- those with malabsorption syndromes, e.g. celiac disease or gastrectomy patients.

RECOMMENDED DIETARY ALLOWANCE

Age	Retinol/Vitamin A (mcg/day)
0-12 months	375
1-3 years	400
4-6 years	500
7-10 years	500
11+ years (male)	1000
11+ years (female)	800
Pregnancy	800
Lactation, 0-6 months	1300
Lactation, 6-12 months	1200

BEST FOOD SOURCES

Food	Retinol (mcg/100g)
halibut liver oil	900,000
lamb's liver	19,900
cod liver oil	18,000
butter	985
margarine	800
cheese, cheddar	363
eggs	190
pig's kidney	160
milk	56
mackerel	45
beef	10
sardines, canned	7

SAFETY

Taken in excess, vitamin A can lead to toxicity because it is stored in the liver. However, it still has a high safety margin in that regular daily intake generally has to exceed 7,500 mcg in women and 9,000 mcg in men before toxic effects are experienced. Vitamin A toxicity is usually fully reversible. The vitamin A intake of pregnant women should not exceed 3,300 mcg per day (from food and supplements combined) unless directed by a health care professional.

INTERACTIONS & CONTRAINDICATIONS

Vitamins A and D (both fat-soluble vitamins) are found together in many food sources, although they are not actually dependent upon one another for their absorption or utilization. A zinc deficiency can affect the function of vitamin A and vice versa. Vitamin A should not be taken with vitamin-A-derived acne medications. The need for vitamin A is decreased if the individual is using the contraceptive pill.

THE B VITAMINS

DESCRIPTION

There are ten different B vitamins that work better when taken together (i.e. synergistically) than when taken separately. This is why the B vitamins are referred to as the B-complex. All the B-complex vitamins are water-soluble, so daily intake of them is required.

THE B–COMPLEX VITAMINS:

- thiamin (B1)
- riboflavin (B2)
- niacin (B3)
- pantothenic acid (B5)
- pyridoxine (B6)
- cobalamin (B12)
- biotin
- folic acid
- choline and inositol

THIAMIN (B1)

DESCRIPTION

Thiamin is known as "the morale vitamin" because of the beneficial effects it has on the nervous system and morale. People with heart disease have been found to have lower than normal levels of thiamin in their heart muscle. Beriberi is a condition, which includes symptoms of general weakness and decreased appetite and was found to be preventable if whole brown rice was eaten instead of refined white rice. In 1926 two doctors isolated the active ingredient missing from the refined grain, which was named thiamin.

Thiamin is a very delicate and easily destroyed vitamin. After vitamin C, it is the least stable of all vitamins. For example, alcohol destroys thiamin. Also, people with a low level of thiamin seem to be troubled more by insects.

Thiamin ensures mental alertness. It is vital for the release of energy from carbohydrates, fats and alcohol, and generally aids digestion. During pregnancy, thiamin ensures the correct growth of the fetus.

DEFICIENCY SYMPTOMS

Severe deficiency is now extremely rare in the Western world, but very low intake leads to beriberi, the symptoms of which include muscle weakness, nausea, loss of appetite and water retention. Minor deficiency of thiamin will lead to mental and emotional problems, such as loss of concentration, memory loss, depression, and irritability. Weight loss and digestive upset may also occur. Probably, the earliest symptom of deficiency is continuous nausea.

THERAPEUTIC USES
- sciatica and low back pain (lumbago)
- deterrence of insects

THOSE WHO MAY NEED TO SUPPLEMENT
- the elderly
- pregnant women
- smokers
- alcoholics
- people under physical or mental stress
- people who have a high carbohydrate intake
- people convalescing from surgery or injury

RECOMMENDED DIETARY ALLOWANCE

Age	Thiamin/Vitamin B1 (mg/day)
0-6 months	0.3
6-12 months	0.4
1-3 years	0.7
4-6 years	0.9
7-10 years	1.0
11-14 years (males)	1.3
15-18 years (males)	1.5
19-24 years (males)	1.5
25-50 years (males)	1.5
51+ years (males)	1.2
11-14 years (female)	1.1
15-18 years (females)	1.1
19-24 years (females)	1.1
25-50 years (females)	1.1
51+ years (females)	1.0
Pregnancy	1.5
Lactation, 0-6 months	1.6
Lactation, 6-12 months	1.6

BEST FOOD SOURCES

Food	Thiamin (mg/100g)
yeast extract	3.1
fortified breakfast cereal	1.8
soya beans, dry	1.10
pork chop	0.57
rice	0.41
bread, whole-meal	0.34
peas, frozen	0.32
peanuts, roasted	0.23
bread, white	0.21
potatoes	0.2
chicken	0.11
beef	0.06
milk	0.05

SAFETY

Thiamin is a very safe vitamin. High dosages of thiamin can be taken for prolonged periods by adults without causing problems. Allergic reactions do sometimes arise when thiamin is injected.

INTERACTIONS & CONTRAINDICATIONS

Thiamin is one of the B-complex vitamins and so ideally should be taken as part of the complex, although single supplementation may be acceptable as part of a nutritional therapeutic program.

RIBOFLAVIN (B2)

DESCRIPTION

Riboflavin is yellow in color and thus has been used as a food-coloring agent. As with all B-complex vitamins, it is water-soluble and requires a regular daily intake. Since it is sensitive to light it must be shielded from light exposure. For instance, milk in glass or clear plastic bottles loses most of its vitamin B2 content if exposed to too much light.

Riboflavin forms two essential coenzymes, flavin dinucleotide and flavin mononucleotide, which together are responsible for converting proteins, fats and sugars into substances that the body can use. Riboflavin is important for healthy skin and hair.

DEFICIENCY SYMPTOMS

Inadequate daily intake of riboflavin may contribute to sores, dermatitis, hair loss, and burning, itching, light-sensitive eyes.

THERAPEUTIC USES

- sores and ulcers
- eye problems
- migraine headaches
- muscle cramps

THOSE WHO MAY NEED TO SUPPLEMENT

- women using the contraceptive pill
- adults with irregular or poor eating habits
- vegetarians, especially vegans

RECOMMENDED DIETARY ALLOWANCE

Age	Riboflavin/Vitamin B2 (mg/day)
0-6 months	0.4
6-12 months	0.5
1-3 years	0.8
4-6 years	1.1
7-10 years	1.2
11-14 years (males)	1.5
15-18 years (males)	1.8
19-24 years (males)	1.7
25-50 years (males)	1.7
51+ years (males)	1.4
11-14 years (female)	1.3
15-18 years (females)	1.3
19-24 years (females)	1.3
25-50 years (females)	1.3
51+ years (females)	1.2
Pregnancy	1.6
Lactation, 0-6 months	1.8
Lactation, 6-12 months	1.7

BEST FOOD SOURCES

Food	Riboflavin (mg/100g)
yeast extract	11.0
lamb's liver	4.64
pig's kidney	2.58
fortified breakfast cereal	1.6
wheat germ	0.61
cheese, cheddar	0.5
eggs	0.47
beef	0.23
milk	0.17
chicken	0.13

SAFETY

Riboflavin is a safe vitamin. No cases of riboflavin poisoning have been recorded. Riboflavin may cause a harmless increased yellow coloration of the urine.

INTERACTIONS & CONTRAINDICATIONS

Riboflavin is one of the B-complex vitamins and so ideally should be taken as part of the complex, although single supplementation is acceptable as part of a nutritional therapeutic program. In this case, it should be taken with brewer's yeast.

NIACIN (B3)

DESCRIPTION

Niacin comes in two forms, an acid (nicotinic acid) and an amide (nicotinamide), neither of which has anything in common with nicotine. Niacin was also referred to as "PP" because it prevented pellagra, a niacin-deficiency disease whose symptoms include diarrhea, dermatitis and dementia. In common with other B vitamins, niacin is water-soluble. In addition to preformed niacin occurring in foods, niacin may also be made in the body from the amino acid tryptophan. Sixty molecules of tryptophan are required to make one molecule of niacin.

The acid form, nicotinic acid, plays an important role in the nervous system and circulation. The amide form, nicotinamide, processes carbohydrates, fats and proteins in the production of energy.

DEFICIENCY SYMPTOMS

These include diarrhea, dermatitis and dementia as seen in pellagra, as well as nervousness.

THERAPEUTIC USES
- improved mobility in arthritis sufferers
- some cases of schizophrenia and alcoholism (megadose supplementation must be under strict medical supervision)
- high blood cholesterol (again, megadose supplementation must be under strict medical supervision)

THOSE WHO MAY NEED TO SUPPLEMENT
- schizophrenics
- alcoholics

RECOMMENDED DIETARY ALLOWANCE

Age	Niacin/Vitamin B3 (mg/day)
0-6 months	5
6-12 months	6
1-3 years	9
4-6 years	12
7-10 years	13
11-14 years (males)	17
15-18 years (males)	20
19-24 years (males)	19
25-50 years (males)	19
51+ years (males)	15
11-14 years (female)	15
15-18 years (females)	15
19-24 years (females)	15
25-50 years (females)	15
51+ years (females)	13
Pregnancy	17
Lactation, 0-6 months	20
Lactation, 6-12 months	20

BEST FOOD SOURCES

Food (mg/100g)	Niacin	Tryptophan	Niacin equivalent*
coffee, instant	24.8	186	27.9
chicken	5.9	221	9.6
beef	4.2	258	8.5
pork chop	4.2	180	7.2
cheese, cheddar	0.1	367	6.2
fish, white	2.9	189	6.0
mung beans, dry	2.0	210	5.5
eggs	0.1	217	3.7
peas, frozen	1.6	58	2.6
bread, whole-meal	4.1**	108	1.8
potatoes	0.6	52	1.5

* The niacin equivalent is the niacin plus the tryptophan contribution in each food source.
** The niacin in whole-meal bread is unavailable to the body; the niacin equivalent figure comes from the tryptophan contribution.

SAFETY

Nicotinic acid can cause facial flushing if taken in large doses. The Health Food Manufacturers' Association therefore recommends the maximum dosage should be 100 mg in an immediate release form and that timed-release nicotinic acid should not be available. Nicotinamide is considered safe up to 2,000 mg/day.

INTERACTIONS & CONTRAINDICATIONS

Niacin works with the other B-complex vitamins, but may be taken separately as part of a nutritional therapeutic program. If taken individually, it should be combined with thiamin and pyridoxine to ensure nervous stability and the conversion of L-tryptophan to nicotinic acid. People suffering from diabetes, gout, stomach ulcers and liver problems should not take nicotinic acid.

PANTOTHENIC ACID (B5)

DESCRIPTION

Pantothenic acid, vitamin B5, is known as B3 in parts of Europe. Its name comes from the Greek panthos, which means "everywhere." It was first isolated from rice husks in 1939. Pantothenic acid is widely found everywhere - in our body tissues and in plants. Pantothenic acid is a B-complex water-soluble vitamin, so a regular daily intake is required.

Pantothenic acid is very important to the process of releasing energy from foods. This is because it is part of coenzyme A, which plays a major role in energy release. Pantothenic acid is used to make and renew body tissues. It is necessary for the production of antibodies and therefore proper immune function.

DEFICIENCY SYMPTOMS

These include fatigue, depression, insomnia, loss of appetite, indigestion, and cramps.

THERAPEUTIC USES

- nausea and indigestion
- premenstrual syndrome (PMS)
- "burning feet" syndrome
- skin disorders

THOSE WHO MAY NEED TO SUPPLEMENT

- alcoholics
- women using the contraceptive pill
- pregnant women
- smokers

REQUIRED NUTRITIONAL INTAKE

There are no specific recommendations regarding the intake of pantothenic acid. An average of 3-7 mg daily is thought to be sufficient for most adults.

BEST FOOD SOURCES

Food	Pantothenic Acid (mg/100g)
brewer's yeast	9.5
pig's liver	6.5
yeast extract	3.8
nuts	2.7
wheat bran	2.4
wheat germ	2.2
eggs	1.8
poultry	1.2

SAFETY

To date, no toxic effects have been recorded with the use of pantothenic acid. It is linked with riboflavin in its function in the production of energy.

INTERACTIONS & CONTRAINDICATIONS

Pantothenic acid is one of the B-complex vitamins and so ideally should be taken as part of the complex, although single supplementation is acceptable as part of a nutritional therapeutic program.

PYRIDOXINE (B6)

DESCRIPTION

Pyridoxine was once known as the "woman's vitamin" because of its beneficial effects in symptoms related to menses. Pyridoxine is a B-complex water-soluble vitamin requiring regular daily intake. Pyridoxine is essential to produce adrenaline (epinephrine) and insulin. Vitamin B6 is reasonably resistant to heat but can be lost from food sources left soaking in water over time. High protein diets increase the need for pyridoxine. Alcoholics typically have low levels of pyridoxine.

Pyridoxine is essential for energy production, necessary for proper functioning of the nervous system, and involved in protein metabolism.

DEFICIENCY SYMPTOMS

Inadequate intake of pyridoxine may cause symptoms of premenstrual syndrome (PMS), lowered white blood cell count, swelling of the abdomen and extremities, and seborrhea (oily skin with crusts and scales) around the eyes, nose and mouth.

THERAPEUTIC USES

- cystitis
- influenza
- conjunctivitis

THOSE WHO MAY NEED TO SUPPLEMENT

- women using the contraceptive pill
- alcoholics
- lactating women
- smokers
- people with heart disease
- women following hormone replacement therapy

RECOMMENDED DIETARY ALLOWANCE

Age	Pyridoxine/Vitamin B6 (mg/day)
0-6 months	0.3
6-12 months	0.6
1-3 years	1.0
4-6 years	1.1
7-10 years	1.4
11-14 years (males)	1.7
15-18 years (males)	2.0
19-24 years (males)	2.0
25-50 years (males)	2.0
51+ years (males)	2.0
11-14 years (female)	1.4
15-18 years (females)	1.5
19-24 years (females)	1.6
25-50 years (females)	1.6
51+ years (females)	1.6
Pregnancy	2.2
Lactation, 0-6 months	2.0
Lactation, 6-12 months	2.0

BEST FOOD SOURCES

Food	Vitamin B6 (mg/100g)
wheat germ	0.95
bananas	0.51
turkey	0.44
chicken	0.29
fish, white	0.29
beef	0.27
brussels sprouts	0.28
potatoes	0.25
bread, whole-meal	0.12
baked beans	0.12
peas, frozen	0.10
bread, white	0.07
oranges	0.06
milk	0.06

SAFETY

Pyridoxine is generally safe to take with no reported cases of toxicity. However, daily doses in excess of 100 mg should be taken under strict medical supervision.

INTERACTIONS & CONTRAINDICATIONS

Pyridoxine is one of the B-complex vitamins and so ideally should be taken as part of the complex, although single supplementation is acceptable as part of a nutritional therapeutic program.

COBALAMIN (B12)

DESCRIPTION

Cobalamin was the last true vitamin to be classified. Vitamin B12 is found in most animal products and some bacteria. Vegetarians and especially vegans can easily become deficient in cobalamin because it is not found in fruits, vegetables, or any other plant sources. Vitamin B12 requires intrinsic factor, secreted by the stomach lining, to be absorbed in the intestines.

Cobalamin helps maintain a healthy nervous system. It maintains the protective "myelin sheath" around the nerves and is used to metabolize fatty acids. Vitamin B12 promotes growth in children and is needed for the production of red blood cells.

DEFICIENCY SYMPTOMS

Inadequate intake or absorption of vitamin B12 can lead to pernicious anemia, which is a deficiency in the red blood cells not related to iron deficiency. If too much folic acid is taken, the symptoms of pernicious anemia may be hidden until irreversible neurological damage has been done and symptoms such as tremors appear. Other symptoms associated with vitamin B12 deficiency include menstrual problems and listlessness.

THERAPEUTIC USES

- moodiness
- paranoia
- mental fatigue and memory impairment
- detoxifying certain chemicals in tobacco smoke

THOSE WHO MAY NEED TO SUPPLEMENT

- vegans and vegetarians
- alcoholics
- pregnant women

- the elderly
- smokers
- those with stomach ulcers
- those taking medications which may injure the stomach lining

RECOMMENDED DIETARY ALLOWANCE

Age	Cobalamin/Vitamin B12 (mg/day)
0-6 months	0.3
6-12 months	0.5
1-3 years	0:7
4-6 years	1.0
7-10 years	1.4
11-14 years (males)	2:0
15-18 years (males)	2.0
19-24 years (males)	2.0
25-50 years (males)	2.0
51+ years (males)	2.0
11-14 years (female)	2:0
15-18 years (females)	2:0
19-24 years (females)	2:0
25-50 years (females)	2:0
51+ years (females)	2:0
Pregnancy	2.2
Lactation, 0-6 months	2.6
Lactation, 6-12 months	2.6

BEST FOOD SOURCES

Food	Vitamin B12 (mcg/100g)
lamb's liver	54.0
pig's liver	23.0
fish, white	2.0
beef, lamb, pork	2.0
fortified breakfast cereal	1.7
eggs	1.7
yeast extract	0.5
milk	0.4

SAFETY

Cobalamin is a very safe vitamin, with injections of as much as 3 mg daily carried out with no side effects.

INTERACTIONS & CONTRAINDICATIONS

Cobalamin is one of the B-complex vitamins and therefore works best synergistically with other B vitamins. However, single supplementation of cobalamin is safe for specific nutritional therapeutic needs. Calcium along with intrinsic factor is required to absorb cobalamin from the intestines.

BIOTIN

DESCRIPTION

Biotin is sometimes referred to as "vitamin H" or "co-enzyme R." It was first discovered as a factor that protected against the toxicity of raw egg whites. It is destroyed when eggs are thoroughly cooked.

Biotin is required in the process of energy production in the cells of the body. It may help prevent premature graying and balding.

DEFICIENCY SYMPTOMS

In adults, inadequate biotin consumption can lead to a scaly dermatitis and hair loss. Deficiency is more commonly seen in infants in whom the scaly dermatitis is described as "cradle cap."

THERAPEUTIC USES

- cradle cap
- dermatitis and eczema
- possible benefit in Candida albicans infections (Candidiasis)

THOSE WHO MAY NEED TO SUPPLEMENT

- pregnant women
- infants suffering from dermatitis and Leiner's disease

REQUIRED NUTRITIONAL INTAKE

The COMA report of 1991 suggested daily intake of biotin from 10 to 200 mcg. The range described is very wide because not enough is yet known about biotin to be more specific. Actual dietary intake of biotin has been found to be between 10 and 58 mcg daily.

BEST FOOD SOURCES

Food	Biotin (mcg/100g)
brewer's yeast	80
pig's kidney	32
yeast extract	27
pig's liver	27
wheat bran	14
wheat germ	12
chicken	10
lamb	6
bread, whole-meal	6
fish, fatty	5

SAFETY

Having been reportedly given to young infants at doses of up to 40 mg without problems, biotin is regarded as a safe vitamin.

INTERACTIONS & CONTRAINDICATIONS

Biotin, as one of the B-complex vitamins, is best taken as part of the group of B vitamins, although single supplementation is safe as part of a nutritional therapeutic program.

FOLIC ACID

DESCRIPTION

Folic acid, or folate, was so named because it is found in green leaves, or foliage. It is sensitive to light, heat and air. Much of it (up to 65 percent) is lost during cooking, and dietary deficiency of folic acid is common. One study showed that 93 percent of men, 98 percent of women aged 18 to 54 years, and 84 percent of women aged over 55 years in the USA are deficient in folic acid.

Folic acid is involved in the formation of healthy cells, being necessary for DNA production and cell division.

DEFICIENCY SYMPTOMS

Inadequate folic acid intake can lead to anemia, for which symptoms include weakness, insomnia, forgetfulness, mental confusion and breathlessness. Folic acid deficiency during pregnancy has been linked to the development of spina bifida in newborns.

THERAPEUTIC USES

- megaloblastic anemia - Folic acid supplementation must be used under strict medical supervision for this treatment, as folic acid can mask pernicious anemia, a vitamin B12 deficiency.

THOSE WHO MAY NEED TO SUPPLEMENT

- pregnant women and women intending to start a family, because the fetus makes large demands on folic acid stores
- celiac disease
- the elderly
- alcoholics

RECOMMMENDED DIETARY ALLOWANCE

Age	Folic acid (mcg/day)
0-6 months	25
6-12 months	35
1-3 years	50
4-6 years	75
7-10 years	100
11-14 years (males)	150
15-18 years (males)	200
19-24 years (males)	200
25-50 years (males)	200
51+ years (males)	200
11-14 years (female)	150
15-18 years (females)	180
19-24 years (females)	180
25-50 years (females)	180
51+ years (females)	180
Pregnancy	400
Lactation, 0-6 months	280
Lactation, 6-12 months	280

BEST FOOD SOURCES

Food	Folic Acid (mcg/100g)
brewer's yeast	2400
wheat germ	310
wheat bran	260
nuts	110
pig's liver	110
leafy green vegetables	90
pulses	80
bread, whole-meal	39
eggs	30
bread, white	27
fish, fatty	26
bananas	22
potatoes	14

SAFETY

Folic acid is generally regarded as having little risk of toxicity in itself, but large doses are to be avoided. This is because large doses of folic acid may mask a vitamin B12 deficiency. For this reason, supplements containing high doses of folic acid are not available.

INTERACTIONS & CONTRAINDICATIONS

As one of the B-complex vitamins, folic acid is best taken with the other B vitamins.

CHOLINE AND INOSITOL

DESCRIPTION

Choline and inositol, members of the B-complex, are both found inside our bodies' cell membranes. Choline increases the production of lecithin, which in turn emulsifies fats. It also helps to control cholesterol.

Inositol plays a role in the response of nerve impulses. Large amounts of inositol are found in men's reproductive organs and semen. It may help prevent eczema, and has been shown to reduce irritability and stress levels. Although considered by some a B vitamin, inositol is not a true vitamin as our bodies can make a small amount of it.

DEFICIENCY SYMPTOMS

Inadequate intake of choline and inositol may contribute to symptoms including mental fatigue and memory impairment, nervousness, eczema, increased blood pressure, and increased susceptibility to colds.

THERAPEUTIC USES

Choline:
- impaired resistance to infection
- angina and thrombosis when taken as lecithin

Inositol:
- nervousness and irritability

THOSE WHO MAY NEED TO SUPPLEMENT
- those with eczema
- individuals suffering from stress and tension
- people with high cholesterol or "hardening of the arteries"

REQUIRED NUTRITIONAL INTAKE

It is recommended that approximately 500-1,000 mg of both choline and inositol be taken daily.

BEST FOOD SOURCES

Food	Choline (mg/100g)	Inositol (mg/100mg)
liver, dessicated	2,170	1,100
heart, beef	1,720	1,600
liver	650	340
beef, steak	600	260
brewer's yeast	300	50
nuts	220	180
pulses	120	160
citrus fruits	85	210
bread, whole-meal	80	100
bananas	44	120

SAFETY

Both choline and inositol are generally safe to take, although very high doses (several grams per day) have been associated with depression.

BETA CAROTENE

DESCRIPTION

Beta carotene is found in the yellow or orange pigment present in many fruits and vegetables. The human body can readily convert beta carotene into vitamin A.

In 1830, the yellow pigment in carrots was isolated and named carotene, however, it was not until 1919 that the connection between carotene and vitamin A was known. It is now known that people with high levels of beta carotene in their diets have less chance of developing certain types of cancers than those with a lower intake of the nutrient. Many studies now show that low intakes of beta carotene are associated with the development of cancer and heart disease. With this in mind, nutrition experts underline the importance of taking five or more good portions of fruits and vegetables daily.

Beta carotene can help to protect the skin from ultraviolet radiation-induced damage and may even protect against skin cancer in the long term. Beta carotene acts as an antioxidant, trapping and neutralizing single oxygen molecules and other free radicals, which can damage the body's cellular membranes, lipids, proteins and vitamins. In addition, beta carotene enhances the immune system by stimulating the activity of interferon.

Cancer, atherosclerosis, diabetes, cataracts, and many other chronic degenerative diseases have been linked to free radical damage. Beta carotene is recognized as a free radical quencher. Numerous epidemiological studies and clinical trials have shown that people who consume high quantities of beta carotene have a lowered incidence of cancer and other chronic diseases. This is in addition to all the functions of vitamin A, to which beta carotene is a precursor.

THOSE WHO MAY NEED TO SUPPLEMENT

- diet is low in carotene-providing fruits and vegetables
- prolonged exposure to bright sunlight
- genetic predisposition or environmental exposure requiring increased protection from free radical damage

REQUIRED NUTRITIONAL INTAKE

As dietary beta carotene contributes to total vitamin A intake, there is not a separate requirement for beta carotene.

Quantities of beta carotene should not be confused with quantities of vitamin A activity. (Only quantities of vitamin A have scientific meaning.) The amount of beta carotene divided by three gives the approximate effective vitamin A activity. So, a 15 mg beta carotene supplement will provide approximately 5 mg of vitamin A.

BEST FOOD SOURCES

Food	Beta Carotene (mcg/100g)
carrots (old)	12,000
spinach	6,000
sweet potato	4,000
apricots, dried	3,600
watercress	3,000
mango	1,200
tomatoes	600
cabbage	300
peas, frozen	300

SAFETY

Beta carotene is a very safe way of getting adequate amounts of vitamin A. At very high levels of beta carotene intake, the body's beta carotene to vitamin A conversion process decreases significantly.

The only known side effect of excess beta carotene intake is "carotenemia," a harmless, fully reversible condition in which the skin turns an orange color.

INTERACTIONS & CONTRAINDICATIONS

Beta carotene cannot be properly converted into vitamin A by diabetics or those with hypothyroidism or severe liver malfunction.

BIOFLAVONOIDS

DESCRIPTION

Bioflavonoids are a group of water-soluble substances that occur mainly as natural pigments in plants, flowers and in citrus fruits (where they are found in the white portion of the peel). They may occur as natural dyes. There have been more than 800 flavonoids discovered to date. The numerous ongoing worldwide bioflavonoid research programs will likely uncover many more to add to the list.

Szent-Gyorgyi, in the mid-1930s, first isolated a material from citrus rind called citrin. It was used in the treatment of weak capillaries (our smallest blood vessels, 1/2000 of an inch in diameter). Citrin was named vitamin P at that time, but soon it was concluded that bioflavonoids were not essential for life and they lost their vitamin status. Although they are no longer considered to belong to the vitamin group, and although most of the world does not use the term 'vitamin P,' some countries, including Russia, still do. Originally, it was thought that flavonoids served no useful role in the prevention or treatment of human disease. Today, we know that although bioflavonoids are not vitamins, they do play a significant role in human nutrition, and in the prevention and treatment of numerous diseases.

Bioflavonoids are active antioxidants. They are present in our food. Their role in the prevention of heart disease is well documented. Some are anticarcinogenic, inhibiting the growth of cancer cells and showing cytotoxic capacity toward certain cancer cells. Bioflavonoids enhance the absorption and effects of vitamin C and have antibacterial potential. They can control the growth of certain bacteria (a bacteriostasic effect) or may actually kill bacteria (an antibiotic effect).

THERAPEUTIC USES

- disorders of blood vessels
- diabetes and its complications
- peptic ulcer disease
- menopausal symptoms
- overexposure to X-rays, or radiation therapy
- thrombophlebitis (blood clot formation, usually in a deep leg vein)

REQUIRED NUTRITIONAL INTAKE

There are no recommended daily requirements for bioflavonoids.

BEST FOOD SOURCES

- citrus fruits (including orange, citron, lemon, lime, grapefruit, and tangerine)
- grapes, cherries, berries, plums, cantaloupes, apricots, papaya
- peppers, broccoli, tomatoes
- tea, coffee, cocoa, red wine

VITAMIN C

DESCRIPTION

Vitamin C is also known as "ascorbic acid," which is the name that appears on food labels. However, its optimum effectiveness and absorption seems to require bioflavonoids. Humans, apes, guinea pigs, and the Indian fruit bat are the only known animal species on our planet that cannot make vitamin C. As a result, we rely on our food and drink to supply us with this vitamin. Vitamin C, one of the antioxidant nutrients, is very delicate. It is water-soluble and sensitive to heat, air and light. Our bodies cannot store it, so a regular daily intake is vital. Since tobacco smoking depletes vitamin C, smokers need a higher daily intake than do non-smokers.

Vitamin C is involved in over 300 biological processes. It seems to be necessary for the effective functioning of the immune system. Vitamin C is required in the production of collagen, the body's intercellular "cement," and speeds healing of wounds and damaged tissues as well as ensuring growth. Additionally, vitamin C allows the body to absorb iron properly and helps change folic acid into a usable form in the body.

DEFICIENCY SYMPTOMS

Significant deficiency of vitamin C leads to scurvy, with symptoms of bleeding gums, muscle and joint aches and pains, dry, scaly skin, irritability, and easy bruising. Some feel that prolonged, marginal deficiency may predispose the individual to cancer and heart disease.

THERAPEUTIC USES

- colds and flu
- following dental treatment
- emotional stress

- alcoholism
- osteoarthritis

THOSE WHO MAY NEED TO SUPPLEMENT
- the elderly
- the ill
- pregnant or lactating women
- athletes
- smokers
- people who drink a lot of alcohol
- recurrent infection
- long term antibiotic, aspirin, contraceptive pill and steroid use

RECOMMENDED DIETARY ALLOWANCE

Age	Vitamin C (mg/day)
0-6 months	30
6-12 months	35
1-3 years	40
4-6 years	45
7-10 years	45
11-14 years (males)	50
15-18 years (males)	60
19-24 years (males)	60
25-50 years (males)	60
51+ years (males)	60
11-14 years (female)	50
15-18 years (females)	60
19-24 years (females)	60
25-50 years (females)	60
51+ years (females)	60
Pregnancy	70
Lactation, 0-6 months	95
Lactation, 6-12 months	95

BEST FOOD SOURCES

Food	Vitamin C (mg/100g)
black currants	200
pepper, green	100
Brussels sprouts	90
mango	80
cauliflower	60
cabbage	55
oranges	50
grapefruit	40
sweet potatoes	25
tomatoes	20
potatoes, new	16
lettuce	15
bananas	10

SAFETY

People with kidney stones should avoid doses of vitamin C over one gram per day and should consult their physician about such use. If you take very high doses (in excess of 5,000 mg) daily, do not stop the dosage suddenly but reduce the amount gradually. Otherwise, this is considered a safe vitamin. Mild diarrhea may result if the body is trying to rid itself of excessive amounts of vitamin C.

INTERACTIONS & CONTRAINDICATIONS

High levels of vitamin C will increase the body's requirement for calcium. Vitamin C may dilute tricyclic antidepressants.

Bioflavonoids increase the activity and absorption of vitamin C. In foods, they always appear naturally with it. Unlike vitamin C, bioflavonoids are relatively stable.

VITAMIN D

DESCRIPTION

Vitamin D is called the "sunshine vitamin." There are two types of vitamin D. Cholecalciferol, or vitamin D3, is found in animal liver oils and is produced in our bodies by the effect of sunlight upon cholesterol-derived substances in the skin. Ergocalciferol, or vitamin D2, is produced when ultraviolet light affects the precursor ergosterol (the "vegetarian" form of vitamin D). Vitamin D is stored in the liver and is fat-soluble. Children need more vitamin D than adults.

In the 17th century, the smog and naturally overcast English weather caused many children to develop rickets (twisted, malformed limbs). Rickets became known as "the English disease."

The most important role played by vitamin D is in bone development. It works by being converted to a hormone, which controls calcium absorption and in turn affects bone development. This is why children have a higher requirement for vitamin D than adults.

Vitamin D is also essential for the development of strong, healthy teeth.

DEFICIENCY SYMPTOMS

In children, rickets ("knock-knees") can develop with inadequate intake of active vitamin D precursors in conjunction with inadequate exposure to ultraviolet radiation. There may be delayed development of teeth and malformation of the limbs with an impairment of posture. In adults, osteomalacia may develop, causing brittle bones, bone pain and muscular spasms.

THERAPEUTIC USES

- prevention and treatment of rickets in children with inadequate exposure to sunlight
- prevention and treatment of osteomalacia in adults

THOSE WHO MAY NEED TO SUPPLEMENT

- vegetarians and vegans, because vitamin D is found mostly in animal products
- elderly or housebound people, who are also unlikely to have sufficient exposure to the sun
- women who have had a series of pregnancies and as a result become short of calcium
- breast-feeding women whose milk may be short of vitamin D, especially during winter

DIETARY REFERENCE INTAKE

Age	Vitamin D (mcg/day)
0-6 months	5
6-12 months	5
1-3 years	5
4-8 years	5
9-13 years (males)	5
14-18 years (males)	5
19-30 years (males)	5
31-50 years (males)	5
51-70 years (males)	10
71+ (males)	10
9-13 years (female)	5
14-18 years (females)	5
19-30 years (females)	5
31-50 years (females)	5
51-70 years (females)	10
71+ years (females)	10
Pregnancy	*
Lactation, 0-6 months	*
Lactation, 6-12 months	*

* Same as other women of same age.

BEST FOOD SOURCES

Food	Vitamin D (mcg/100g)
cod liver oil	212.5
herring and kipper	22.4
salmon, canned	12.5
milk, evaporated	4.0
eggs	1.6
butter	0.8
liver	0.82
cheese, cheddar	0.3
milk, whole*	0.03
milk, skimmed*	0

*unfortified

SAFETY

Vitamin D may have the highest potential of toxicity of all the vitamins, so care must be taken not to exceed the recommended guidelines. However, vitamin D is safe up to five times the recommended amount. Too much vitamin D may have a deleterious effect on the kidneys, heart and lungs.

INTERACTIONS & CONTRAINDICATIONS

Vitamin D is important for the absorption of calcium and phosphate. Although vitamins A and D are often found together, they are not, in fact, co-dependent. Some cardiac drugs when taken with vitamin D may cause irregular heart rhythm, so consult your medical doctor for appropriate supervision.

VITAMIN E
(TOCOPHEROL)

DESCRIPTION

Vitamin E is one of the antioxidant nutrients (other vitamins include A and C, and minerals include selenium and zinc). Vitamin E has had many names, one of the earliest was "the anti-sterility vitamin." Vitamin E is fat-soluble and exists naturally in many different forms and strengths.

Vitamin E is a powerful antioxidant, protecting the body's cells and important nutrients and aiding the healing process. It helps break down fats, increasing oxygen efficiency and thus increasing fitness. Vitamin E is felt by many to be vital for proper nervous system function. It has been used to treat menopausal hot flashes because it regulates the body's temperature, prevent thrombosis (blood clots), and help maintain healthy skin.

DEFICIENCY SYMPTOMS

Deficiency of vitamin E is unlikely as it is easily and widely available. There is no problem if fats and oils can be absorbed properly, but some conditions may lead to a shortage of vitamin E because of impaired absorption. Chronic shortage of this vitamin is thought to lead to a host of illnesses. Such conditions include low red blood cell count, cirrhosis of the liver, alcoholism, celiac disease, and cystic fibrosis.

THOSE WHO MAY NEED TO SUPPLEMENT

- women with menstrual or menopausal problems
- postoperative patients
- people with poor circulation or varicose veins
- sufferers of Parkinson's disease
- people with cardiovascular problems

RECOMMENDED DIETARY ALLOWANCE

Age	Vitamin E (a-TE mg/day)
0-6 months	3
6-12 months	4
1-3 years	6
4-6 years	7
7-10 years	7
11-14 years (males)	10
15-18 years (males)	10
19-24 years (males)	10
25-50 years (males)	10
51+ years (males)	10
11-14 years (female)	8
15-18 years (females)	8
19-24 years (females)	8
25-50 years (females)	8
51+ years (females)	8
Pregnancy	10
Lactation, 0-6 months	12
Lactation, 6-12 months	11

BEST FOOD SOURCES

Food	Vitamin E (mg/100g)
wheat germ oil	178
safflower oil	97
sunflower seeds, raw	74
sunflower oil	73
almonds	37
mayonnaise	19
wheat germ	17
margarine, hard	16
peanut butter	9
soybean oil	8

SAFETY

Vitamin E is thought to be safe up to 3,200 mg per day. High dosages have occasionally been associated with fatigue, nausea, raised blood pressure and mild gastrointestinal problems. These symptoms are reversible with a gradual decrease of vitamin E intake.

INTERACTIONS & CONTRAINDICATIONS

If one is taking anticoagulant medicines, vitamin E must only be taken with a physician's approval. Vitamin E activity is increased by selenium and vice versa. Diabetics are generally advised to avoid vitamin E supplements.

VITAMIN K

DESCRIPTION

Vitamin K is found in fatty foods. Nature has provided enough fats in foods containing fat-soluble vitamins to ensure their absorption without eating additional fat. Vitamin K is stored in the liver. High doses of fat-soluble vitamin K taken over a long period of time may be toxic for some people. A normal supplemental dose is 300 to 500 mcg.

Vitamin K is necessary for the formation of a chemical required in blood clotting. The body cannot manufacture vitamin K although it is produced by the intestinal flora. Green leafy vegetables and chlorophyll, either liquid or tablets, are a good source of vitamin K.

DEFICIENCY SYMPTOMS

A vitamin K deficiency may occur if there is a lack of bile, which is necessary for the absorption of all fat-soluble vitamins. Sprue (celiac disease) and colitis cause poor absorption of vitamin K in the intestines. A deficiency may cause diarrhea, miscarriage, nosebleeds and hemorrhages anywhere in the body.

RECOMMENDED DIETARY ALLOWANCE

Age	Vitamin K (mcg/day)
0-6 months	5
6-12 months	10
1-3 years	15
4-6 years	20
7-10 years	30
11-14 years (males)	45
15-18 years (males)	65
19-24 years (males)	70
25-50 years (males)	80

INTERACTIONS & CONTRAINDICATIONS

Large doses of synthetic vitamin K can cause a toxic reaction. Anyone on anticoagulation therapy such as warfarin must consult his or her medical professional before even considering vitamin K as it can reverse the anticoagulant's action.

PABA

DESCRIPTION

The full name of PABA is Para-aminobenzoic acid. Although regarded by some as the newest addition to the B-complex group of vitamins, it is actually a part of folic acid. PABA is essential for friendly bacteria to grow and has been suggested to have a cosmetic value, possibly retarding graying of the hair.

The role of PABA is not yet fully explored, but it is thought to be helpful for the metabolism of red blood cells and amino acids, as well as for healthy skin.

DEFICIENCY SYMPTOMS

Because the action of PABA is not yet fully known, deficiency symptoms are also not known.

THERAPEUTIC USES

- vitiligo (condition characterized by depigmentation of the skin)
- scleroderma and lupus erythematosus, two severe skin disorders

REQUIRED NUTRITIONAL INTAKE

As yet there are no official guidelines regarding the daily intake of PABA.

BEST FOOD SOURCES

Not many specifics have been recorded about the amount of PABA in individual foods. However, liver, eggs, wheat germ and molasses are known to be good sources.

SAFETY

PABA is best taken with the other B vitamins but can be taken on its own if required. Dosages in excess of 8 g daily may result in constant itching and, more seriously, liver problems.

INTERACTIONS & CONTRAINDICATIONS

None have been reported to date. However, the dosages used in clinical trials for the treatment of scleroderma and lupus erythematosus were extremely high and should not be self-administered.

INDEX
OF
MINERALS

BORON

DESCRIPTION

Boron is a mineral, which only recently has been recognized as playing a part in human nutrition. Its exact functions have yet to be discovered. It is believed to be important in maintaining bone density, and thought to have particular relevance to women.

Administered to menopausal women, it slowed the rate of calcium and magnesium losses and doubled levels of an estrogen metabolite, which is responsible for retaining calcium in the bone. It is thought to help broken bones heal faster. It has been reported to diminish symptoms of rheumatoid arthritis.

DEFICIENCY SYMPTOMS

No specific symptoms have been recognized with regard to boron deficiency as yet, although a shortage of boron in animals has been documented, resulting in stunted growth.

REQUIRED NUTRITIONAL INTAKE

Since boron has yet to be defined as essential for life, there is no definitive recommended nutritional intake.

BEST FOOD SOURCES

Food	Boron (mg/100g)
soy	2.8
prunes	2.7
raisins	2.5
almonds	2.3
rose hips	1.9
peanuts	1.8
hazelnuts	1.6
dates	0.92

wine .... up to 0.85

honey 0.72

SAFETY

As little as 100 mg may produce toxic effects. Short-term doses up to 9 mg are usually safe, but advice from your health care practitioner should be sought out. Vomiting and diarrhea are typical symptoms of boron toxicity.

Boron in the form of boric acid may be quite toxic if ingested or inhaled. The body absorbs boron in too large a quantity in this way. The situation is exacerbated if it is applied to broken skin or membranes.

INTERACTIONS & CONTRAINDICATIONS

If boron is lost as a result of osteoporosis, extra calcium seems to make up for the loss. Animal studies have shown that a deficiency of vitamin D increases the need for boron.

CALCIUM

DESCRIPTION

Calcium is the most abundant mineral in the human body. Over 1.5 percent of the body's total weight is calcium, found in the skeletal and other tissues. To be absorbed, cobalamin (vitamin B12) needs calcium. Calcium needs vitamin D in order to be absorbed. We rely on our food and drink to supply us with calcium, as our bodies cannot make it. Adults lose 400-600 mg of calcium daily.

Osteoporosis is a major problem for many people, primarily in post-menopausal women. In this condition, there is a decrease in the actual bone mass. Often, falls and other accidents can lead to fractures of the hip, vertebrae, wrist, or other parts of the body. Almost all health care professionals agree that nutrition is the key to the avoidance of osteoporosis. It is generally recognized that osteoporosis is related to a deficiency of calcium, throughout the individual's life span. The calcium supplementation needed should begin long before any symptoms of brittle bones are obvious, and should be guided by a physician or nutritionist.

Calcium is a mineral, which is often not easily assimilated by the body and may be in short supply due to dietary restrictions. Besides the normal food sources of calcium, such as dairy products and certain grains and vegetables, there are many calcium supplements available. These include calcium lactate, calcium phosphate, calcium gluconate, calcium carbonate, chelated calcium, and dolomite. Some nutritionists advise the taking of several different forms of calcium to assure proper assimilation. It is also essential that vitamins D and C be taken along with calcium for maximum absorption. Many nutritionists will also recommend magnesium to balance the calcium intake, although no specific ratio is universally agreed upon.

Another major problem is the excessive use of phosphoric acid, which may leach calcium out of the bones. Phosphoric acid can be readily found in many of the cola-type beverages on the market today. The use of such products should be limited. Some nutritionists feel that extra dietary phosphorus is beneficial, but this phosphorus is not in the form of phosphoric acid. This can be found in poultry, eggs, meat, fish, seeds, nuts, and whole grains.

Another element, which appears to play a role in osteoporosis, is silicon (silica), which must be taken in a natural, organic, water-soluble form to be absorbed. It appears that silica may help keep calcium in the bone structure, and if it is lacking, calcium may tend to "leak out" of the bones. Aside from ready made nutritional sources of silica or silicon, some good natural sources are rice hulls, wheat bran, soybean meal, and citrus pectin. There is also some evidence that in women, high doses of citrus bioflavonoids (1,000 mg/day) have a mild estrogenic effect, which may be beneficial in preventing the calcium loss of osteoporosis.

The element fluorine, which tends to make bones harder, may also play a role in the treatment of osteoporosis. Some physicians are using large doses of this element by prescription in severe cases of this ailment. It must be emphasized that this procedure is considered experimental and remains controversial. Nutritionists feel that fluorine in modest doses (not in the form of sodium fluoride as is found in most water supplies) may be helpful in osteoporosis. Certain sea foods and some plants contain fluorine in organic form, and may be beneficial to individuals with osteoporosis.

Weight bearing appears to be necessary in order to retain calcium in the bones. Astronauts, especially when exposed to long periods of time in space, lose a large amount of calcium from their bones. This is apparently due to the significant decrease of bearing weight through their bones, which is similarly seen in patients following prolonged bedrest. Such prolonged exposures in a weightless environment may present an opportunity for experimentation with various nutritional supplements to see if calcium loss can be prevented.

In addition to its important role in the skeleton, calcium also strengthens teeth. It is required in the process of the clotting of blood. Calcium is also necessary for the proper function of the nervous system and muscular contraction.

DEFICIENCY SYMPTOMS

Inadequate calcium intake can lead to a number of symptoms including muscle spasm, mental confusion, and abdominal pain. Chronically inadequate intake of calcium increases the risk of osteoporosis, which increases susceptibility to bone fractures.

THERAPEUTIC USES

- periodontal disease- reduction of bone density where teeth are rooted
- high blood pressure (anecdotally reported)

THOSE WHO MAY NEED TO SUPPLEMENT

- pregnant and lactating women
- post-menopausal women
- people who regularly take antacids
- vegans

DIETARY REFERENCE INTAKE

Age	Calcium (mg/day)
0-6 months	210
6-12 months	270
1-3 years	500
4-8 years	800
9-13 years (males)	1300

14-18 years (males) 1300
19-30 years (males) 1000
31-50 years (males) 1000
51-70 years (males) 1200
71+ (males) 1200
9-13 years (female)....................................... 1300
14-18 years (females) 1300
19-30 years (females) 1000
31-50 years (females) 1000
51-70 years (females) 1200
71+ years (females)....................................... 1200
Pregnancy .... *
Lactation, 0-6 months...................................... *
Lactation, 6-12 months.................................... *

* Same as other women of same age.

BEST FOOD SOURCES

Food	Calcium (mg/100g)
skimmed milk, powder	1,230
cheese, cheddar	800
sardines	550
tofu	506
dried figs	280
evaporated milk	260
watercress	220
natural yogurt	200
milk	103
peanuts, roasted	61
cabbage	57
bread, whole-meal	54
eggs	52
fish, white	22

SAFETY

Calcium is safe to take even in large amounts, since the body rids itself of unwanted quantities. However, consult with your healthcare professional if you are predisposed to forming kidney stones or other similar problems.

INTERACTIONS & CONTRAINDICATIONS

Calcium acts synergistically with vitamin D, which is needed for calcium absorption. It seems to be inversely related to magnesium and potassium, in that low levels of one produce high levels of the other. It is best to avoid excessive amounts of potassium, which can lower calcium levels.

CHROMIUM

DESCRIPTION

Chromium is a mineral that is essential for human health. It is an essential cofactor for the hormone insulin, which regulates the metabolism of protein, fats and carbohydrates. Chromium is particularly involved in the metabolism of carbohydrates. Because of this, it can be a deterrent to the onset of diabetes. Chromium also helps maintain an appropriate blood pressure. Individuals tend to retain less chromium as they age.

DEFICIENCY SYMPTOMS

Deficiency symptoms include high blood sugar and/or cholesterol levels, and poor tolerance of glucose.

THOSE WHO MAY NEED TO SUPPLEMENT

- people predisposed to diabetes
- people needing to lower total cholesterol levels and increase HDL levels
- athletes wanting to develop lean muscle

REQUIRED NUTRITIONAL INTAKE

The National Research Council has tentatively recommended 50 to 200 mcg of chromium as an "adequate" daily amount. The Food and Drug Administration has proposed 130 mcg as its Reference Daily Intake. Nutritional researchers find that doses of 200 to 400 mcg produce significant health benefits. There is no specific required nutritional intake value for chromium as given by the COMA report, but a daily amount in excess of 25 mcg is thought to be adequate and safe.

BEST FOOD SOURCES

Food	Chromium (mg/100g)
egg yolk	183
molasses	121
brewer's yeast	117
beef	57
cheese	56
grape juice	47
bread, whole-meal	42
wheat bran	38
raw sugar	35
honey	29
potatoes, old	27
wheat germ	23
chicken leg	18
spaghetti	15
spinach	10
bananas	10
haddock	7
milk, skimmed	2

INTERACTIONS & CONTRAINDICATIONS

Chelated zinc has been reported to sometimes act as a substitute for chromium.

COPPER

DESCRIPTION

Copper is involved in many bodily processes, such as production of melanin (affecting the color of skin and hair), and the production of superoxide dismutase (SOD), which protects against free radicals and cell damage. Copper appears to be necessary for proper transmission of nerve impulses in the nervous system, energy production, oxidation of fatty acids, and transference of oxygen in the muscles.

Seventy percent of copper content is lost when flour is refined. Copper has been used in contraceptive devices because it is toxic to sperm.

DEFICIENCY SYMPTOMS

In infants, copper deficiency may result in pale skin, diarrhea and dilated veins. In adults, falling white blood count and anemia may be found. Some reports indicate there may be a diminishing sense of taste. Theoretically, there may be an increased risk of heart disease.

THERAPEUTIC USES
- joint pain in osteoarthritis

THOSE WHO MAY NEED TO SUPPLEMENT
- individuals taking a zinc supplement (zinc depletes copper reserves)
- those with Menke's syndrome (a rare, genetic disease)

REQUIRED NUTRITIONAL INTAKE

Age	Copper (mg/day)
9-12 months	0.3
1-3 years	0.4
4-6 years	0.6
7-10 years	0.7
11-14 years	0.8
15-16 years	1.0
18+ years	1.2
Lactation	1.5

BEST FOOD SOURCES

Food	Copper (mg/100g)
oysters	7.6
whelks	7.2
lamb's liver	6.0
crab	4.8
brewer's yeast	3.3
olives	1.6
hazelnuts	1.4
shrimps	0.8
cod	0.6
bread, whole-meal	0.25

SAFETY

Toxicity is rarely observed, although this may be because copper is usually not found as an individual supplement by itself. Daily intake of up to 10 mg is generally safe, but it is strongly advised not to exceed this amount (FAQ/WHO Expert Committee, 1971).

INTERACTIONS & CONTRAINDICATIONS

As mentioned above, zinc depletes copper. Vitamin A requires copper and other nutrients to be absorbed. Vitamin C improves copper absorption.

GERMANIUM

DESCRIPTION

Organic germanium, bis-carboxyethyl germanium sesqui-oxide (or "Ge-132"), has been tested in the treatment of a wide variety of medical problems that require improved oxygenation and immune function. Found in high quantities in garlic, Siberian ginseng, reishi (lingzhi) mushroom, and other medicinal plants, germanium has been shown to enhance gamma-interferon and activate macrophages and natural killer cells. Several Japanese medical studies have reported beneficial effects in malignancies and rheumatoid arthritis. Additional research studies have indicated that germanium has immunomodulating properties and may also function as a free radical scavenger. Germanium appears to be a natural regulator of homeostasis, found to be nontoxic even at high oral doses.

TOXICITY

Not known

IRON

DESCRIPTION

Iron is found in two different forms in food. "Heme" iron is exclusive to animal, fish and fowl. "Non-heme" iron is found in fruits and vegetables.

The world's most common vitamin/mineral deficiency is of iron (World Health Organization). Although iron is plentiful in the planet and vital for humans, it exists in very small amounts in our bodies, only about 4-5 grams.

Iron is a vital ingredient of the blood pigment, hemoglobin. It is important in the production and release of energy, helps to keep our immune systems working properly, and helps young children to grow.

DEFICIENCY SYMPTOMS

With iron deficiency anemia, individuals may feel fatigue, have a pale face, and have white rather than a more normal pink color to the membranes of the eyes and fingernails. If allowed to progress, later symptoms such as dizziness, abnormally fast heart rate, loss of appetite, and insomnia may develop. Sometimes, inadequate iron may cause pruritis (generalized itching all over the body).

In early childhood, iron deficiency may cause stunted growth and impaired mental abilities.

THERAPEUTIC USES
- iron deficiency anemia
- pruritis (itching)
- mental disability in young children

THOSE WHO MAY NEED TO SUPPLEMENT
- women of childbearing age because of menstrual blood loss
- vegetarians

- the elderly
- pregnant women and lactating women
- adolescents
- athletes
- alcoholics

REQUIRED NUTRITIONAL INTAKE

Age	Iron (mg/day)
0-3 months	1.7
4-6 months	4.3
7-12 months	7.8
1-3 years	6.9
4-6 years	6.1
7-10 years	8.7
11-18 years (males)	11.3
11-50 years (females)	14.8
19-50 years (males)	8.7
50+ years	8.7

BEST FOOD SOURCES

Food	Iron (mg/100g)
curry powder	29.6
fortified breakfast cereal	16.7
lamb's liver	7.5
pig's kidney	6.4
apricots, dried	4.1
bread, whole-meal	2.7
corned beef	2.4
chocolate, plain	2.4
eggs	2.0
beef	1.9
watercress	1.6
bread, white	1.6
cabbage	0.6
red wine	0.5
fish, white	0.5
potatoes	0.4

SAFETY

Some people cannot tolerate large amounts of supplemental iron. Large doses of supplemental iron should not be given to children. However, toxicity is not commonly found.

INTERACTIONS & CONTRAINDICATIONS

Vitamin C improves absorption of heme iron (animal, fish or fowl origin). Copper is needed to turn iron into hemoglobin (used in the production of red blood cells).

MAGNESIUM

DESCRIPTION

Magnesium is one of the most abundant minerals in the human body, following calcium and phosphorus. Half of the body's magnesium is found in bones, the rest is in the body's other tissues. Magnesium is necessary for proper muscle and nerve function, energy release, growth (e.g. reproduction of DNA), and to maintain healthy cells and tissues. Magnesium is also needed for proper endocrine (hormonal) function. It may also have a protective effect on the heart.

DEFICIENCY SYMPTOMS

Inadequate magnesium may adversely affect many functions of the body. Symptoms of magnesium deficiency include irritability, tension and stress, muscle tremors and cramps, parethesias ("pins and needles"), and arrhythmia (irregular heartbeat). A deficiency of magnesium may be related to a shortage of potassium.

THERAPEUTIC USES
- PMS
- muscle spasms and resulting pain
- possibly angina (cardiac pain) and arrythmia

THOSE WHO MAY NEED TO SUPPLEMENT
- women suffering from PMS
- alcoholics
- people taking diuretics

DIETARY REFERENCE INTAKE

Age	Magnesium (mg/day)
0-6 months	30
6-12 months	75
1-3 years	80
4-8 years	130
9-13 years (males)	240
14-18 years (males)	410
19-30 years (males)	400
31-50 years (males)	420
51-70 years (males)	420
71+ (males)	420
9-13 years (female)	240
14-18 years (females)	360
19-30 years (females)	310
31-50 years (females)	320
51-70 years (females)	320
71+ years (females)	320
Pregnancy	per age +40
Lactation, 0-6 months	*
Lactation, 6-12 months	*

* Same as other women of same age.

BEST FOOD SOURCES

Food	Magnesium (mg/100g)
peanuts, roasted	180
sunflower seeds	129
bread, whole-meal	76
cheese, cheddar	25
fish, white	23
chicken	21
beef, steak	18
potatoes	17
oranges	13
eggs	12

SAFETY

Magnesium is safe to take even in large doses, except for people with kidney problems or when otherwise contraindicated.

INTERACTIONS & CONTRAINDICATIONS

Magnesium and calcium utilization in many bodily functions are interconnected and therefore their ratio in our diet should be between 1:1 and 1:2.

MANGANESE

DESCRIPTION

Manganese is a trace mineral, which we therefore cannot make ourselves but must obtain from our food and drink. Manganese promotes healthy function of the nervous system and ensures bones develop correctly and remain healthy. Manganese is present in women's sex hormones. Eighty-six percent of manganese content is lost when flour is refined. Eighty-nine percent of manganese is lost when sugar is refined.

DEFICIENCY SYMPTOMS

Since manganese deficiency has only been observed in one person, it is impossible to describe the symptoms of its deficiency. However, in animals, a lack of manganese results in problems with reproduction, stunted growth, and deformed offspring.

REQUIRED NUTRITIONAL INTAKE

The COMA, USRDA and US/Canadian DRI do not give a required nutritional intake for manganese, but a safe minimal intake per day is given at "above 1.4 mg daily for adults."

BEST FOOD SOURCES

Food	Manganese (mg/100g)
bread, whole-meal	4.3
wheat germ	4.2
avocados	4.2
chestnuts	3.7
hazelnuts	3.5
sunflower seeds	2.1
peas	2.0

almonds 1.9
tea (1cup) 1.5
coconut 1.3
pineapple 1.1
plums 1.0
lettuce 0.7
bananas 0.6
beet root 0.6
watercress 0.5

SAFETY

Manganese supplements taken by mouth have not been reported to produce toxicity to date. Too much manganese in children has been associated with learning disorders.

INTERACTIONS & CONTRAINDICATIONS

Manganese is thought to increase the effect of iron when red blood cells are produced.

MOLYBDENUM

DESCRIPTION

Molybdenum is a trace mineral, the dietary importance of which is only beginning to be known. Its presence in the diet depends mainly on the soil in which vegetables and other edible produce are grown. When plants are grown in molybdenum-poor soil, they lack that essential mineral. An example of this was observed in Lin Xian, in China's Hunan Province, where there was an extraordinarily high incidence of esophageal carcinoma occurring over many generations. When molybdenum was added to the soil, the rate of this deadly disease declined. It is speculated that the cancer was not caused by molybdenum deficiency. Rather, nitrosamines produced in the food were not being metabolized properly due to a deficiency in the plants' root systems of the molybdenum-requiring enzyme, nitrate reductase. The nitrosamines were felt to be the direct cause of the cancer.

Nitrates and nitrites are found in various lunch meats and sausages. Consumption of them can lead to the formation of carcinogenic nitrosamines in the stomach. In addition to vitamin C, supplemental molybdenum can help reduce nitrosamine levels. Unless one is confident that he or she is eating plenty of produce grown in molybdenum-rich soil, taking a mineral supplement containing this essential trace element is highly advisable. Soil deficiencies of molybdenum are widespread and common, and processing of flour and sugar eliminate it completely.

Molybdenum is required for correct function of xanthine oxidase, an enzyme responsible for iron metabolism. It is required for the production of uric acid, a waste product found in the blood and urine. Molybdenum helps to detoxify excess copper and helps ensure normal sexual function in men.

DEFICIENCY SYMPTOMS

As mentioned above, lack of molybdenum may appear as male sexual dysfunction.

THOSE WHO MAY NEED TO SUPPLEMENT

- individuals with proven molybdenum deficiency
- those with excess blood copper levels

REQUIRED NUTRITIONAL INTAKE

The COMA report does not set a required nutritional intake for molybdenum, but states that a safe intake is "between 50 mcg and 400 mcg."

BEST FOOD SOURCES

Food	Molybdenum (mcg/100g)
canned beans	350
wheat germ	200
liver	200
lentils	120
sunflower seeds	103
kidney beans	75
green beans	66
macaroni	51
eggs	50
rice	47
noodles	45
chicken	40
bread, whole-meal	26
potatoes	25
shell fish	20
apricots	14

SAFETY

Oversupply of molybdenum can lead to toxicity, so its consumption should be kept within the range of 150-500 mcg for adults and 50-300 mcg for children.

POTASSIUM

DESCRIPTION

Most of our potassium is within the cells themselves, especially inside the skeletal muscles. The small amount of potassium that is outside of our cells helps maintain the correct amount of water in our cells. Generally, potassium functions in conjunction with sodium, helping maintain proper acid-base balance and ensuring the normal transmission of nerve impulses and muscle contraction. It therefore is necessary for proper peristaltic movement in the intestines.

DEFICIENCY SYMPTOMS

Inadequate potassium may produce symptoms including restlessness, loss of appetite, nausea, thirst, and drowsiness.

THERAPEUTIC USES

- with use of potassium-depleting medications (diuretics) for high blood pressure
- night cramps

THOSE WHO MAY NEED TO SUPPLEMENT

- people taking potassium-depleting diuretics (taken under medical supervision)
- people taking antibiotics on a long-term basis (those that deplete stores of potassium, again with medical advice)
- athletes or physical laborers (who can lose potassium through sweat)

REQUIRED NUTRITIONAL INTAKE

Age	Potassium (mg/day)
0-3 months	800
4-6 months	850
7-12 months	700
1-3 years	800
4-6 years	1,100
7-10 years	2,000
11-14 years	3,100
15+ years	3,500

BEST FOOD SOURCES

Food	Potassium (mg/100g)	Sodium (mg/100g)
instant coffee	3,780	81
potato crisps	1,190	550
raisins	860	52
sunflower seeds, unsalted	850	3
potatoes	360	8
pork	360	65
cauliflower	350	8
tomatoes	290	3
chicken	290	75
bread, whole-meal	230	560
peas, frozen	190	3
streaky bacon	183	1,245
oranges	180	2
milk, whole	140	50

SAFETY

High intake of potassium can cause problems in people with kidney disease, which could result in heart failure. One should take potassium supplements under a doctor's supervision, especially when taking a potassium-depleting medication. Generally it is better to get one's daily potassium needs from a well-balanced diet.

INTERACTIONS & CONTRAINDICATIONS

Sodium and potassium usually are used in concert in the body to maintain correct fluid and electrolyte balance. Therefore, a high salt intake may increase the requirement for potassium.

SELENIUM

DESCRIPTION

Selenium, an essential trace mineral, derives its name from the goddess of the moon, Selene. Before 1979, it was thought that selenium was important only for animals, and poisonous to humans. Now it is known to be an antioxidant, which is 50 to 100 times more powerful than vitamin E and essential for humans. As an antioxidant, like vitamins C and E, it destroys potentially harmful free radicals. It maintains a healthy heart and normal liver function, ensures correct functioning of the eyes, is necessary for healthy hair and skin, and may help to protect against cancer.

DEFICIENCY SYMPTOMS

Selenium deficiency is fairly rare in the West while we continue to enjoy foods from other countries whose soil is still rich in selenium. For this reason specific deficiency symptoms relating to selenium are not documented. However, Keshan disease (a heart disease which primarily affects Chinese children) does arise when dietary intake of selenium is inadequate.

THERAPEUTIC USES

- arthritic symptoms
- high blood pressure
- skin, hair and nail problems
- helps detoxify the body of heavy metals (e.g., mercury in dental fillings)

THOSE WHO MAY NEED TO SUPPLEMENT

- individuals who may not be eating properly
- vegetarians
- the elderly

- smokers
- pregnant women and nursing mothers

RECOMMENDED DIETARY ALLOWANCE

Age	Selenium (mcg/day)
0-6 months	10
6-12 months	15
1-3 years	20
4-6 years	20
7-10 years	30
11-14 years (males)	40
15-18 years (males)	50
19-24 years (males)	70
25-50 years (males)	70
51+ years (males)	70
11-14 years (female)	45
15-18 years (females)	50
19-24 years (females)	55
25-50 years (females)	55
51+ years (females)	55
Pregnancy	65
Lactation, 0-6 months	75
Lactation, 6-12 months	75

BEST FOOD SOURCES

Food	Selenium (mcg/100g)
organ meats (kidney, liver, heart)	approx. 40
fish and shellfish	approx. 32
meat	approx. 18
whole grains and cereals	approx. 12
dairy products	approx. 5
fruits and vegetables	approx. 2

SAFETY

Extremely high doses of selenium (5,000 mcg per day) taken over a long period of time have resulted in hair loss and deformed fingernails. Daily doses of 1,000 mcg over a long period of time have resulted in the sweat smelling of garlic despite the fact that no garlic was eaten, as well as thicker but weaker fingernails. Diarrhea, nausea, fatigue and irritability are other symptoms experienced with excessive daily doses.

INTERACTIONS & CONTRAINDICATIONS

Selenium works with vitamin E as an antioxidant, and may be helpful in certain heart diseases. Selenium in conjunction with vitamins C and E has inhibited cancer in laboratory studies with animals.

ZINC

DESCRIPTION
Zinc is a trace mineral. Only 2-3 grams are found in the adult body. However, it is a component of over 80 enzymes, which means that it has more functions than any other trace mineral. This includes keeping nails, skin and hair healthy and maintaining the reproductive organs in both men and women.

DEFICIENCY SYMPTOMS
Lack of adequate amounts of zinc in the body can result in white flecks in the nails, acne, eczema and psoriasis. There can be lowered immune function causing increased susceptibility to infections.

THERAPEUTIC USES
- rheumatoid arthritis, as zinc and essential fatty acids are functionally linked
- the common cold (zinc and vitamin C combine to strengthen the immune system)
- prostate problems
- adolescent acne (found in many acne creams)
- athletes foot (found in many foot powders)

THOSE WHO MAY NEED TO SUPPLEMENT
- pregnant women (zinc is necessary for fetal development)
- vegetarians (legumes and grains may bind zinc, which is then not absorbed by the body)

RECOMMENDED DIETARY ALLOWANCE

Age	Zinc (mg/day)
0-6 months	5
6-12 months	5
1-3 years	10
4-6 years	10
7-10 years	10
11-14 years (males)	15
15-18 years (males)	15
19-24 years (males)	15
25-50 years (males)	15
51+ years (males)	15
11-14 years (female)	12
15-18 years (females)	12
19-24 years (females)	12
25-50 years (females)	12
51+ years (females)	12
Pregnancy	15
Lactation, 0-6 months	19
Lactation, 6-12 months	16

BEST FOOD SOURCES

Food	Zinc (mg/100g)
cheese, cheddar	4.0
beef, steak	3.8
bread, whole-meal	1.8
eggs	1.5
chicken	1.1
bread, white	0.6
milk	0.4
fish, white	0.4
potatoes, old	0.3

SAFETY

Excess doses of zinc (150-450 mg daily) have been shown to cause low blood cell counts. Two thousand mg of zinc per day can cause vomiting and gastrointestinal upset. Doses of 18.5 mg daily can reduce blood copper levels but no physical symptoms have been reported. Daily doses of 15 mg of zinc are considered to be a safe upper limit beyond which one should seek medical advice.

INTERACTIONS & CONTRAINDICATIONS

Zinc is required to release vitamin A from the liver. High zinc intake reduces levels of copper and iron, while high iron intake can reduce zinc levels, as can high amounts of cadmium.

INDEX OF DIETARY SUPPLEMENTS

ANDROSTENEDIONE

DESCRIPTION

When it comes to "drug free" testosterone boosters, one effective natural substance is the adrenal hormone, androstenedione. A step removed from DHEA, it is the direct precursor to testosterone. It is produced naturally in both men and women. Surprisingly, it is also found in the pollen of the Scotch pine tree, from which it has been manufactured as a dietary supplement. In reasonable amounts taken orally, the liver will convert it to testosterone. Androstenedione could be the most controversial supplement of the decade, and there is much talk of it in gyms around the world.

Androstenedione was first isolated in 1935. However, it was not fully investigated until the late 1950's, when scientists determined androstenedione is converted in the body to testosterone and vice versa. There are two different pathways in the body that can create androstenedione: either from DHEA or from a hormone called 17 alphahydroxyprogesterone. One study quoted in a German patent application (DE 42 14 953 A1) stated that oral doses of androstenedione, given to men at levels of 50 mg and 100 mg raised testosterone levels 140 percent to 183 percent and 211 percent to 237 percent, respectively.

Although there is some research showing it causes a significant surge of serum testosterone as well as sustained levels, there are no studies documenting increases in muscle mass. The East German scientist, Oettel, studied the effects of androgens on the central nervous system and how enhanced neuron firing improves athletic performance. He felt that twice-a-day "pulses" of testosterone increased the performance of athletes.

Conversely, a study done in 1989 suggested that a regular once-a-day testosterone pulse is effective. Researchers compared two groups of laboratory animals. One group got a large dose of testosterone each day. The other received the same milligram total, spread throughout the day in smaller doses. The single dose increased muscle mass more than the smaller, frequent dose schedule.

Administering testosterone in a single once a day pulse is a new idea. There may be fewer side effects with a single delivery. It is possible that by spiking one's natural testosterone levels only once or even twice a day may keep the body from lowering its natural production of testosterone. This has been found to be a problem that occurs with anabolic steroid use.

With the exception of professional football, androstenedione has not been banned in any other drug-tested sports. The International Olympic Committee has added DHEA, but not androstenedione to its prohibited-substance list. Even though the testosterone/epitestosterone ratio may rise to 14:1 during the day of androstenedione use, it could fall below 6:1 (within the passing range) the day after stopping its use.

Is using androstenedione cheating? By itself, androstenedione is not a muscle builder. Like DHEA, it only works if and when it is converted to testosterone in the body. You might say this supplement "upgrades" the body's natural production of testosterone.

Blood test results for dosages higher than 100 mg of androstenedione taken orally are not available. If a 100 mg dose can produce a greater than 200 percent increase in serum testosterone, can a 200 mg dose produce a 400 percent increase? This simply is not known.

For a strength boost, a dose 60 minutes before training could produce favorable results. After an oral dose, testosterone levels peak at about 60 minutes.

TOXICITY, CAUTIONS & CONTRAINDICATIONS

Since androstenedione seems to cause a brief burst of testosterone, it may or may not cause any of the usual testosterone side effects including acne, prostate hypertrophy, and a decrease in HDL cholesterol. It should not be used by anyone with known health problems without first consulting a physician. It is not advisable for women to use this supplement, as it may cause acne, facial hair growth, and a lowering of the voice. It is not a drug and thus it does not pose the same health risks as anabolic steroids, such as liver toxicity and problems with the kidneys.

ALPHA LIPOIC ACID

DESCRIPTION

Alpha lipoic acid is an antioxidant that prevents free radical damage. Although there have been hundreds of studies over the past 40 years revealing how lipoic acid energizes metabolism, the new excitement about this vitamin-like substance can be seen in many recent studies focusing on how it improves the physique, combats free radicals, protects our genetic materials, slows aging, and may help protect against heart disease and cancer.

Alpha lipoic acid has been used for nearly 30 years in Europe for both insulin-dependent and non-insulin-dependent diabetic patients. It has been used to treat diabetic neuropathy, help regulate blood sugar, and prevent diabetic retinopathy and cardiopathy. Lipoic acid not only helps protect but also may help regenerate nerves. Lipoic acid has been used for decades to protect the liver and detoxify the body of excess metals such as iron and copper, and heavy metal pollutants such as cadmium, lead and mercury. Recent studies have suggested that lipoic acid appears to help slow the progression of HIV infection to clinical AIDS. It is being studied in the treatment of Parkinson's disease and Alzheimer's disease.

Lipoic acid is both water- and fat-soluble and is an important antioxidant helping protect the body against damage that can contribute to heart disease, cancer, aging and many other health problems. The damage is caused by free radicals, which are the undesirable byproducts of metabolism. Lipoic acid also restores the activity levels of the enzymes glutathione peroxidase, catalase, and ascorbate free radical reductase. It appears that alpha lipoic acid, alone or together with vitamins C and E, is an effective treatment for radiation exposure, lessening incidents of oxidative damage and normalizing organ function.

Although our bodies produce small amounts of lipoic

acid, it is usually not enough. We rely on foods such as potatoes and red meat to supply additional amounts for optimal health. Alpha lipoic acid supplements are now available in health food stores.

RECOMMENDED DOSE:
50 – 200 mg a day (hypoglycemic patients should take alpha lipoic acid in divided doses)

TOXICITY, CAUTIONS & CONTRAINDICATIONS
Not known

BACILLUS LATEROSPORUS

DESCRIPTION

Bacillus laterosporus is a naturally occurring single cell organism. It is found in the inner lining of the stomach and intestinal tract as a natural "friendly" bacteria. Bacillus laterosporus has been used to treat a number of maladies, including Candidial infection, chronic fatigue, and digestive problems. It is non-toxic and non-allergenic. Most Bacillus laterosporus is passed on to humans through foods we eat. At least, that's the way it was before chemical farming was introduced.

Discovered in a remote part of Iceland, Bacillus laterosporus in the soil was found to contribute to the growth of enormous, vibrant-colored, rich-tasting vegetables. Those who ate vegetables grown in this type of soil not only received beneficial nutrients, they also consumed large quantities of the friendly bacteria themselves.

Similar to Lactobacillus acidophilus, Bacillus laterosporus produces unique metabolites with antibiotic, anti-tumor and immune modulating activity. Resistant to stomach acids, Bacillus laterosporus helps maintain a proper balance of friendly bacteria in the intestines, thereby maintaining good colon health. Similar to Lactobacillus bifidus and acidophilus, it helps to bolster the digestive process through the removal of yeast, fungi and other pathogens, thus maintaining a predominance of "good" intestinal flora.

Bacillus laterosporus is one of the best supplements a person can take to restore optimal digestive function. It has been tested in independent laboratories and has been shown to be beneficial in Candida albicans, Salmonella, Streptococcus faecalis, and Escherichia coli infections.

TOXICITY, CAUTIONS & CONTRAINDICATIONS

No known toxicity

BEE PRODUCTS
• BEE POLLEN
• ROYAL JELLY
• PROPOLIS

DESCRIPTION

Pollen is the male component of the plant reproductive system and is produced in flower blossoms. It is gathered by bees, mixed with the bees' own digestive enzymes, and carried back to the hive in the "pollen baskets" on their hind legs. Bee pollen is a complete and natural food. In fact, bee pollen is the only food that contains all essential nutrients necessary to sustain life, including vitamins, minerals, trace elements, proteins, carbohydrates, fats, amino acids, antibiotics, enzymes, and hormones.

For centuries people in every land have had similar beliefs regarding the miraculous power of bee pollen. Some claims are that it improves energy level, aids digestion, relieves allergy symptoms and bronchial disorders, improves regularity, creates muscular vigor, improves prostate problems, rejuvenates skin, and combats the side effects of chemotherapy treatments. Additionally it has been used as an aphrodisiac.

Bee pollen in North America is considered to be most potent nutritionally when gathered from herbal sources in high desert regions, which have naturally low humidity and usually are relatively free from industrial pollutants and pesticides. A special pollen trap that prevents rodent contamination ensures its purity.

As it comes from the hive, bee pollen has an outer husk that is usually not digested by the human body. However, a process has been developed that cracks or breaks this husk of the bee pollen grains, which enables the vital nutrients to be easily digested. This is a cold process, which avoids the destruction of vital enzymes.

THERAPEUTIC USES
- frequent infections
- hormone imbalance
- hypertension
- prostate diseases
- nervous and endocrine system complaints
- also used for sore throats, acne, fatigue, sexual problems, and allergies

TOXICITY, CAUTIONS & CONTRAINDICATIONS
Bee pollen must be avoided by those allergic to bee stings or other bee products.

ROYAL JELLY

DESCRIPTION

In the larval stage, there is no difference between queen, worker, and drone bees. In the first two days of life, each bee larva is fed a special "milk" which a nurse bee secretes from a gland in its head. This secretion is called "royal jelly." It is so potent that in two days the larvae change into little bees, and are then taken off royal jelly and fed a diet of honey and pollen. However, the bee chosen to be the next "queen" continues to be fed only royal jelly. Now something extraordinary takes place. This chosen queen grows into a female considerably larger in size than ordinary bees. She lives 40 times longer, and is capable of laying up to 2,000 eggs per day, which is 2 and 1/2 times her own weight!

An analysis of royal jelly shows that it is packed with nutrients. Most of the B vitamins are present (thiamin, riboflavin, nicotinic acid, biotin, inositol, folic acid, pyridoxine, cobalamin, and pantothenic acid) as is vitamin C. The minerals found include calcium, magnesium, phosphorus, sodium, potassium, iron, manganese, zinc and cobalt. Other nutrients include amino acids (the building blocks of protein), sugars, fatty acids, hormones and nucleotides (nucleic acids).

Research shows that royal jelly stimulates the adrenal glands and produces an increase in the body's metabolic rate. This may be responsible for the reports of increased energy, enhanced sexual capabilities, and increased appetite.

Royal jelly is the richest source of natural acetylcholine, the important neurotransmitter that allows many of the nerve endings in the brain to transmit nerve impulses from one nerve fiber to another. It is acetylcholine that has been found to be deficient in the tangled bundles of nerve endings in patients with Alzheimer's disease. This helps explain the most significant symptom in this affliction, memory loss.

In addition, royal jelly is very rich in biotin and nucleic acids, the latter making up the DNA of each cell's chromosomes. In combination, these nutrients help promote cell tissue regeneration. There still remain a small percentage of components in royal jelly that have not as yet been identified. Royal jelly maintains its highest potency when suspended in natural honey.

THERAPEUTIC USES
- acne and allergies
- arthritis
- constipation, weight loss, and anorexia
- vascular diseases and angina
- menstrual problems
- conditions associated with the aging process (reportedly helps enhance energy and vitality and to increase stamina)
- anxiety
- ulcers

TOXICITY, CAUTIONS & CONTRAINDICATIONS
Royal jelly must be avoided by those allergic to bee stings or other bee products.

PROPOLIS

DESCRIPTION

Certain trees exude a resinous sap from their buds and bark which has antibiotic qualities to protect that tree. It is collected by bees and metabolized with their own secretions. Propolis contains a complex of biologically active vitamins, minerals, and enzymes along with a unique range of flavonoids or cell building components.

Propolis, the name given to this substance by the ancient Greeks, means "defense before the city." They believed propolis was used by the bees to defend their hive (city) against bacteria and intruders. For instance, if an intruder such as a mouse enters the hive, it will be stung to death and then covered with propolis. Normally the decaying process would cause serious bacterial contamination. However, the propolis-mummified mouse remains embalmed, preventing contamination.

Antibacterial and antiviral properties found in propolis work to raise the body's natural resistance to disease by stimulating the immune system. Unlike prescription antibiotics, propolis does not kill the friendly bacteria in the digestive system, which are necessary for the body to synthesize certain B vitamins as well as vitamin K. Use of antibiotics can contribute to a deficiency of these important vitamins.

A strong immune system is the key to protection against disease and infection, cellular destruction and aging. The nutritional activity of propolis has been proven to rejuvenate the immune system. It is effective in helping to deal with a wide variety of illnesses including ulcers, colds, flu, hypertension, and skin conditions.

TOXICITY, CAUTIONS & CONTRAINDICATIONS

Propolis must be avoided by those allergic to bee stings or other bee products.

BETA GLUCAN

DESCRIPTION

Beta-1, 3-D-glucan is a polysaccharide, which naturally occurs in the cell walls of organisms such as common baker's yeast. It triggers an immune response in the body, creating a systemic defense against viral, bacterial, fungal, parasitic and possibly certain neoplastic invaders. It also has potent antioxidant and free radical scavenging capabilities and may be a cholesterol-lowering agent.

Beta glucan works by activating or turning on macrophages in the body. Macrophages are the "sentries" of the immune system. These cells, normally resting, circulate throughout the body. Upon introduction of a foreign body (antigen), they become "activated" and initiate a whole cascade of immunological events. These events include: secretion of interleukin 1 (lL1), which induces T cells to aggressively attack the foreign matter; secretion of complement proteins, which destroy foreign cells by punching holes in their membranes; secretion of hydrolytic enzymes, which promote an inflammatory response; secretion of alpha-interferon (INF-a), which activates cellular genes resulting in the production of proteins that confer an antiviral state on the cell; tumor necrosis factor-alpha (TNF-a), which directly kills tumor cells; and secretion of interleukin-6 and granulocyte stimulating factors, which promote formation and development of red and white blood cells.

In addition to all the above, the activated macrophage plays an important role in the immune response by literally ingesting (via phagocytosis) and degrading the foreign material. This not only has the obvious benefit of clearing the antigen but, during this process, the macrophage uses the parts of the invader to "present" them to T-cells, which are the most aggressive components of the immune response.

The result is an amplified immune system response until the viral and/or other invaders are defeated. When a single dose is administered, the macrophage activity will peak in 72 hours; 72 hours later, the activity level returns to the previous plateau.

Supplementing with beta -1, 3-D-glucan will benefit people with impaired immunity from any cause. This includes those who are susceptible to infectious disease (as in advanced HIV infection), patients undergoing radiation or chemotherapy, people over 40 years of age whose immune systems begin to slow down, individuals with poor nutrition or who consume chemically preserved food, those under mental or emotional stress, athletes and others who work out extensively, and those with a high risk of cardiovascular disease.

Studies have reported a 25-27 percent infectious complication rate in patients undergoing major surgery with an average cost per infected patient of $12,000. The efficacy of beta glucan in the prevention of sepsis has been demonstrated for both gram-negative and gram-positive bacteria. With an average dosage being 30-100 mg/kg/day the financial benefits are obvious (doses have been tested to 1000 mg/kg/day with no noted side effects).

THERAPEUTIC USES
- Klebsiella pneumoniae, Staphylococcus aureus, and other infections
- accelerates wound repair and decreases postoperative infection
- Escherichia coli-induced peritonitis
- tumor reduction
- enhances survival in leukemic animals
- possible anti-melanoma properties
- reported to increase the rate of repopulation of the immune system after irradiation

BROMELAIN

DESCRIPTION

Bromelain is an enzyme derived from pineapple juice. It curdles milk and lyses protein molecules (i.e. a proteolytic enzyme). Bromelain is a powerful anti-inflammatory and inhibits platelet aggregation, dissolving fibrin clots. Oral administration of the enzymes bromelain, papain or amylase, or combinations of them, induces synthesis of anticancer compounds called cytokines (tumor necrosis factor-alpha, interleukin-1 beta and interleukin-6) in human peripheral blood mononuclear cells when first incubated out of the body with interferon-gamma. Similar results were obtained in vitro, applying all of the compounds simultaneously.

THERAPEUTIC USES

- poor digestion of protein
- inflammation and edema due to injury or surgery, especially following episiotomy
- inflammation and edema in chronic conditions such as osteoarthritis
- possible use in cancer therapy, especially in combination with interferon-gamma

TOXICITY, CAUTIONS & CONTRAINDICATIONS

Bromelain is contraindicated in the presence of gastric ulcers or gastrointestinal irritation. It can cause allergic reactions and skin irritation, but no other toxicity has been reported.

CETYL MYRISTOLEATE

DESCRIPTION

Arthritis, the number one chronic illness in the US, affects 37 million Americans in all age groups. One person in seven suffers from it. Conventional medicine offers many medications to treat arthritis, including corticosteroids and non-steroidal anti-inflammatory drugs, both of which are capable of producing complications including kidney and liver damage as well as gastric irritation or ulceration. A rarely mentioned side effect of conventional medications is the inhibition of cartilage repair, resulting in an actual worsening of the arthritic condition. Occasionally, patients die from these drugs. When one weighs risks against benefits, it is questionable whether the prescription drugs are any better than common aspirin. Because of the seriousness of drug side effects, it is always good news when a natural product shows promise in helping arthritis sufferers. One such product is cetyl myristoleate, a new and unique natural compound which is being hailed as a significant nutritional breakthrough.

Cetyl myristoleate (CM or CMO) is described as an ester of a fatty acid which appears to function in three ways: as a lubricant, benefiting muscles and other tissues making them more pliable; as an immune system modulator, benefiting autoimmune diseases such as lupus, rheumatoid arthritis, and multiple sclerosis; and as an anti-inflammatory agent.

Discovered in 1962 by Harry W. Diehl, a researcher from the National Institutes of Health, interest in CMO grew out of the observation that certain strains of mice are completely immune to arthritis (just as sharks rarely develop cancer). Two years later a substance unique to mice was finally identified and isolated, which turned out to be the fatty acid compound now known as cetyl myristoleate. The next step was to see if CMO could prevent arthritis in other animals, and tests on rats proved it could. Commercial development by drug companies following these discoveries was impeded by the fact that CMO is a natural substance and not patentable as a drug.

Like anything else, CMO does not work 100 percent of the time. Best results are obtained when it is part of a comprehensive program, which includes other appropriate nutritional supplements and dietary measures such as restriction of animal fat, sugar, alcohol, citrus juices and caffeine, as well as liver detoxification.

TOXICITY, CAUTIONS & CONTRAINDICATIONS

Thousands of people have taken CMO with no known adverse side effects. Occasionally, people experience belching as they may with fish oils. Until further studies can be done, pregnant or lactating women should not take CMO. People with asthma or a history of severe allergic reactions should only take CMO under medical supervision.

CHITOSAN (CHITIN)

DESCRIPTION

Chitosan is derived from a substance called chitin, which is present in the exoskeleton of insects and shell-fish. It is generally harvested from the shells of crabs and is a polymer of N-acetyl glucosamine. Chitosan absorbs five times its weight in fat, cholesterol, and bile acids in the gastrointestinal tract. It reduces serum cholesterol with no side effects.

Chitosan is different from most fibers in that its particles have a positive electric charge, which attracts negatively charged fat molecules. Thus, by absorbing fat and holding these fats in the digestive tract, the body does not have the building blocks of cholesterol and cholesterol production is reduced. Depending upon the amount of chitosan taken, it is possible for it to absorb over one-third of our dietary fat. The resulting indigestible mass is then eliminated.

As with all fibers, lots of fluid, typically eight glasses daily, should be taken for best results. Other natural fibers do not have the same capacity to bind with lipids or fats in the intestine, but simply increase bulk and absorb water to help maintain proper elimination of waste through the colon. Chitosan itself is calorie free and is, therefore, very useful as a dietary supplement to assist those wishing to decrease dietary fat absorption and possibly lose weight, yet maintain a low calorie, high-fiber diet.

It is well documented that obesity is one of the main causes of premature death in the Western world. Most experts agree that exercise combined with a low-fat, high-fiber diet will help improve and maintain health and overcome obesity. Fortunately, science has discovered that chitin will absorb more fat than other dietary fibers and thus reduce the amount of fat deposited in the body.

One of the most effective and widely used cholesterol lowering drugs today is Cholestyramine. Though effective, this drug has been linked to colon cancer and damage to the liver and intestinal cells. In comparative studies, chitosan lowered the cholesterol almost as effectively as Cholestyramine but without the side effects.

THERAPEUTIC USES
- weight loss
- cholesterol reduction

TOXICITY, CAUTIONS & CONTRAINDICATIONS
Chitosan appears to be non-toxic and well tolerated, with absolutely no side effects when used as directed. No studies as yet have reported on the possible binding effects of chitosan on essential fatty acids or fat-soluble vitamins. It is suggested that those supplements be taken at a different time than the chitosan.

CHLORELLA

DESCRIPTION

Chlorella is a microscopic two-billion-year-old algal plant. It is nutrient dense and is easily digestible after processing has broken the cell walls. Chlorella is approximately 58 to 60 percent protein with a complete amino acid profile. It is a rich source of chlorophyll, vitamins, minerals, and many phytochemicals. It is especially high in beta carotene, iron and zinc. Chlorella is also an excellent source of vitamin B12 for vegetarians.

Few products in recent years have gained as much attention as has this microscopic, unicellular relative of sea kelp. Numerous animal studies have demonstrated the anti-tumor and antiviral activities of chlorella, as well as its interferon-inducing effects. Significant research has also been done on chlorella growth factor (CGF), which is a liquid extract from the nucleus of the algae cell containing proteins, vitamins, carbohydrates and nucleic acids. Many reports and clinical trials have shown anti-tumor activity against a variety of cancers, both in humans and animals. Anti-tumor activity has been observed specifically against breast cancer, leukemia, ascitic sarcoma and liver cancer.

Chlorella has been shown to have immune-enhancing effects, and to have antiviral activity against cytomegalovirus in mice and equine encephalitis virus in horses. Antihypertensive and antihyperlipidemic activities were observed with a protein fraction derived from chlorella.

Chlorella has the highest chlorophyll content of any known plant - five to ten times as much as spirulina, wheatgrass or barleygrass. Chlorella's cell wall has been shown to help eliminate toxins, pesticides, and heavy metals from the body by binding to them in the digestive tract. It also induces interferon production, which is important to immune system function. Because of chlorella's abundance of beta carotene, it may aid in the prevention of certain cancers.

THERAPEUTIC USES
- whole food protein source
- enhance immune response and liver function
- increases resistance to colds and viruses
- possible anti-tumor effects
- heavy metal toxicity in humans
- powerful cleanser of the blood stream, bowels and internal organs
- Japanese studies have shown that chlorella and CGF increase the growth rate, improve degenerative disease, and lower blood pressure and cholesterol

TOXICITY, CAUTIONS & CONTRAINDICATIONS
No known toxicity.

CHONDROITIN SULFATE

DESCRIPTION

Chondroitin sulfate (CS) is a glycosaminoglycan, which is found naturally in the body and is important in maintaining elasticity and integrity of many types of body tissues, including connective tissue and the walls of blood vessels. CS is a component of cartilage, which in turn is a component of connective tissue. Helping to give support and shape to tissues, cartilage is found in joints, between vertebrae and elsewhere. CS creates a net electronegative charge, which attracts water. Hydration maintains the compressibility, elasticity, fluidity, and joint movement characteristic of healthy cartilage.

As a result of aging, the water content of cartilage decreases, causing problems in joint mobility. The integrity and function of cartilage can also be detrimentally affected by acute traumatic injury, arthritis, malnutrition and other conditions. CS is also a component of the walls of blood vessels and is therefore important in maintaining vascular health. In addition, CS is known to activate lipoprotein lipase on capillary endothelial cells, which helps blood lipids to be metabolized. Studies have demonstrated the effectiveness of CS supplementation for the healing of connective and certain other tissues that have been injured or otherwise degraded through malnutrition, aging or certain drugs and diseases. CS supplementation may also be indicated as a preventative or possible treatment agent for certain vascular conditions.

THERAPEUTIC USES

- helps restore and maintain connective tissue
- improves fluidity of joint movement
- improves and maintains vascular health

TOXICITY, CAUTIONS & CONTRAINDICATIONS

Chondroitin sulfate is considered to be safe and there are no known contraindications. Usual dosage is two 300 mg capsules taken two to three times per day during the healing phase. One to two 300 mg capsules, one to three times daily, may be used as a maintenance dose.

CHROMIUM PICOLINATE

DESCRIPTION

Chromium is a mineral that is essential for human health. The National Research Council has tentatively recommended 50 to 200 micrograms of chromium as an "adequate" daily amount. The Food and Drug Administration has proposed 130 micrograms as its Reference Daily Intake. Nutritional researchers find 200 to 400 micrograms produce significant physique enhancement and other health benefits. Chromium is an essential cofactor for the hormone insulin, which regulates the metabolism of protein, fats and carbohydrates - practically everything we eat.

Chromium picolinate is an exceptionally bioavailable organic form of this vital nutrient. It provides chromium in the nutritional trivalent form and is extremely safe. Extensive studies on chromium picolinate with humans and animals during the past several years have produced no adverse effects. Very high levels of chromium picolinate given to laboratory animals over a short period of time also showed no adverse effects. Lifetime feeding of chromium picolinate to rats increased their life span by 25 percent.

Chromium deficiency can be very serious. It is clearly a risk factor for Type II diabetes (non-insulin dependent diabetes) and is also a factor in cardiovascular disease. Fat gain and lack of energy may also result from inadequate amounts of chromium.

The trace mineral chromium is vital to health yet is undersupplied in modern diets. It is more likely to be in short supply than any other nutrient. Even diets devised by competent nutritionists rarely supply the minimum recommended amounts. Most people are deficient in chromium partly because chromium is not essential for plants, which can thrive without chromium. That means that humans cannot rely on getting adequate amounts from their diet. Food processing removes much of the naturally occurring chromium, and refined sugar consumption further depletes what little chromium we do get. U.S. Department of Agriculture studies show there is so little chromium in foods that you would need to consume about 14,000 calories daily to get 200 micrograms of chromium.

How chromium picolinate assists in fat reduction is not yet clear. Rodent studies show that insulin works in the brain to increase calorie burning (thermogenesis) while curbing food intake. If chromium picolinate aids some of these insulin actions in the brain, a reduction of body fat could be anticipated. However, further clinical studies will be required to clarify the mechanisms by which chromium picolinate promotes a leaner human physique.

Recent studies show that at least one in four adults has reduced sensitivity to insulin. The majority of these people do not become diabetic because the pancreas compensates by secreting increased amounts of insulin. In these people, insulin insensitivity is a "silent" problem. There is increasing evidence that this "silent" insulin insensitivity is, in fact, a serious medical problem and a risk factor for cardiovascular disease.

COENZYME Q10

DESCRIPTION

Coenzyme Q10 (CoQ10) occurs naturally in all human cells. It is essential in cellular energy production. CoQ10 is made in the body, but production is reduced as we get older. It is also found in foods (especially meat), but cooking and processing methods tend to destroy it. The Japanese have been using supplemental CoQ10 for many years but it was not until 1974 that pure CoQ10 was obtained in large enough quantities for the Japanese to initiate organized trials on patients.

THERAPEUTIC USES

- reduce risk of heart disease, including congestive heart failure, ischemic heart disease, and irregular heartbeat
- periodontal (gum) disease
- obesity when due to a CoQ10 deficiency
- restore energy
- improve immunity -stimulates antibody formation

TOXICITY, CAUTIONS & CONTRAINDICATIONS

CoQ10 is usually effective at levels of 15-60 mg per day but over 100 mg has been used without any toxicity problems or side effects. There are no known drug interactions or other contraindications for CoQ10.

COLLAGEN

DESCRIPTION

For ages, people have searched for a way to fight the aging process. Cleopatra swore by ewe's milk baths. In the 1940's, Hollywood stars used hemorrhoid cream on their skin. More recently, people have taken injections of embryonic fluids as a way of restoring a youthful, wrinkle-free appearance. The word "collagen" is derived from kolla, the Greek word for glue. It is the strong fiber that weaves throughout the lower layers in your skin, providing the strength and support your skin needs to fight wrinkles. As one ages, the body's ability to make collagen diminishes. The quality of collagen in skin, hair, nails, bones and teeth gradually weakens. Soon the collagen fibers lose their moist texture and become rigid. Once that happens, free radicals attach to the collagen strands, making them thick and unyielding. While collagen on the inside is weakened and damaged by free radicals, on the outside the skin is becoming wrinkled, nails are becoming ridged and brittle, and hair is becoming dull and thin.

Part of the natural aging process is related to amino acid levels. No matter how diligent one is regarding diet, ordinary foods and vitamins cannot produce the special amino acids which collagen supplies. Today, although there are many sources of collagen as an effective moisturizing ingredient in creams, a new product has been developed which is the only FDA-classified collagen food supplement that fights the aging process. These hydrolyzed collagen supplements are available as chewable wafers and tablets. They help give the body the raw materials it needs to repair its own collagen supply. In doing so, they help fight the natural aging process.

THERAPEUTIC USES

- grow, repair and maintain healthy skin, bones, muscles, tendons, cartilage, gums, teeth, eyes and blood vessels
- repair damaged nails
- slow down hair loss
- thicken hair diameter up to 45 percent

COLLOIDAL SILVER

DESCRIPTION

Silver has been used as a disinfectant since ancient times. Today there is some dispute about what form of silver is safest and most effective. There has been insufficient data to resolve the issues. Colloidal silver, developed in the 1800's, consists of fine particles suspended in a liquid and is felt by many to be the safest and most effective form for oral use. It is yellow-gold in color, and because of refraction it has a cloudy appearance when light passes through it, so that a cone shape appears inside. The closer to yellow-gold the color is, the finer the particle size. Particles can be suspended electrically, though at least the larger particles will soon settle out, leading most suppliers to bind the particles in egg albumin to keep them in suspension longer. It is supplied in de-ionized water with no additives, in a sealed container that does not attract the particles. However, there are some authorities that feel chelated silver bound to peptides or other proteins is the least toxic and most effective form.

Colloidal silver is lethal to most microorganisms. It is apparently taken into their cell membranes, interfering with cell "respiration." The best-documented use of colloidal silver is for prevention and control of bacteria and fungi, both internal and external. It is effective against so many bacteria, it is simpler to list those against which it is known or likely to be ineffective: Citrobacter freundii, Enterobacteriaceae (some strains), Klebsiella pneumoniae, Proteus mirabilis, Enterobacter cloaceae, Escherichia coli (some strains), P. stutzeri (some strains), vegetative B. cereus spores, B. subtilis, and bacteria selected and specially preconditioned for use in silver mining operations. It has been found to be effective against the fungi Candida albicans, C. globata, and M. furfur, among others. It has also been used to promote bone healing when applied to the site using electrical current, as described in the reference below.

Colloidal silver is absorbed directly into the bloodstream through the mucous membranes of the mouth, esophagus, stomach, and small intestine. Taken in small amounts, it usually does not adversely affect the colonies of friendly bacteria in the large intestine. One source says that true colloidal silver tends to accumulate in the tissues, giving residual benefits after use is discontinued, but does not cause discolored areas as does prolonged intake of high amount of larger silver particles.

THERAPEUTIC USES
- bacterial infections
- other infections, such as yeast infection

TOXICITY, CAUTIONS & CONTRAINDICATIONS

If colloidal silver reaches the large intestine and disrupts the friendly flora there, Lactobacillus acidophilus and bifidus or Bacillus lactosporus supplementation to restore the proper balance is advisable. Colloidal silver may be toxic to the body's own cells; not enough is known at this time to ensure safety of all forms. Use sparingly and with caution.

COLOSTRUM

DESCRIPTION

Colostrum is a pure and natural product resulting from collecting and drying (under strict government regulated protocols) the milk obtained within the first six hours after birth of a calf. Colostrum is collected from selected herds and processed to meet all good manufacturing practices (GMP) of the USDA for a biological ingredient. Colostrum is made during the last two months of pregnancy at which time the cow starts lactating. This initiates the biochemical processes which result in the super concentrated immune proteins for the new calf. The cow produces more than is required, and it is this overflow that is harvested. To obtain the most potent colostrum, it should be collected in the first six to 36 hours.

Colostrum is rich in immune proteins classified as immunoglobulins (IgG, IgA, and IgM), which is produced to provide the newborn with these antibodies from the mother's immune system. The newborn's immune system is not yet fully functioning and colostrum provides antibodies required to ward off and defend against infections such as bacterial, viral, and fungal, and other antigens.

The implication for individuals experiencing the effects of a compromised immune system is that colostrum would be a logical whole food supplement. Additionally, there are many vitamins in high concentrations along with rich sources of minerals in easily assimilated forms. Recent research has proven the existence of IGF-1 (insulin like growth factor) which is of interest to athletes. Colostrum also contains a small molecular weight moiety called transfer factor, which is a messenger to the immune system preparing it for defense against specific antigens. This can be a very promising way to offer health benefits through an oral supplement as it is small enough to be absorbed through the digestive system. The "probiotic" functions of colostrum are well researched, and effectiveness against various gastrointestinal problems - such as diarrhea, etc. - is well established.

For any person wishing to supplement his or her diet and to be assured of receiving the factors provided in colostrum, daily supplementation of 500 to 1,000 mg is recommended during the initial stage of intake, and a twice-weekly dose of like amounts is recommended for maintenance. This can be in a protein powder drink, capsule or tablet, depending on preference. The probiotic functions can be combined with synergistic organisms such as Lactobacillus bifidus and Bacillus lactosporus., resulting in a product with dual approaches to normalizing the bowel environment. Future colostrum applications are being developed combining clinical research and product processing.

Colostrum has many more components than whey concentrate, which is often sold as colostral whey - a misnomer.

CORDYCEPS MUSHROOM

DESCRIPTION

According to traditional Chinese medicine, the Kidneys are responsible for the origin of life, storing the life essence. If the Kidneys are strengthened, the life essence is increased, and thus one is full of vigor and vitality and can live a long and healthy life. Cordyceps mushroom (Cordyceps sinensis), is a high-quality, natural nutrient, used in traditional Chinese medicine especially to nourish the Kidneys and yin energy and to moisturize the lung. Its ingredients include cordycepin, which benefits the Kidneys and strengthens the body to cure all kinds of consumptive diseases. The classic "Questions and Answers on A Hundred Medical Herbs" says, "Cordyceps sinensis is a panacea." From the viewpoint of modern medicine, a quarter of the blood pumped out from the heart flows through the kidneys, and metabolites and other residue are thus filtered. Therefore, through functions of filtration, secretion and reabsorption, the kidneys play an important role in regulating, promoting and steadying various systems in the body, such as blood circulation, water metabolism and respiration. Any damage or disease in the kidneys is harmful to health. The kidneys are very important in many life activities.

According to modern medicine, in the blood plasma of a sufferer of chronic renal failure, the leucine, isoleucine, trytophan, tyrosine and lysine in the free amino acids drop drastically, leading to malnutrition, edema and weakness. Cordyceps, however, contains these amino acids. Supplementation with Cordyceps provides the essential amino acids needed by the patient.

TOXICITY, CAUTIONS & CONTRAINDICATIONS

Cordyceps sinensis is a pure, natural product, neither toxic nor having side effects. It can safely be taken over a long period of time.

CREATINE

DESCRIPTION

There has been a great deal of excitement among athletes about the dietary supplement creatine. Scientific research has verified that creatine is not just an energy source that powers muscle tissue. Creatine is becoming the athlete's most important supplement because it increases muscle strength, promotes significant increases in muscle fiber size and muscle cell volume (lean mass) without increasing body fat or water content, increases muscle energy per unit time, and improves performance during both short-duration high-intensity as well as intermittent activities.

Creatine helps accelerate energy recovery between bouts of intense exercise. For example, after a sprint, the next sprint would be easier and at a greater speed with regular creatine supplementation. It may reduce fatigue by reducing lactic acid build-up in short-burst and other exercises. It permits more intense training, which further improves strength and muscle growth by delaying muscle fatigue. Creatine regenerates ATP-energy to increase muscle-working time in anaerobic activity such as in training to failure. It also helps spare muscle fiber degradation, allowing more work with less catabolism.

Creatine is made in our bodies. Ninety-five to 98% of the body's creatine is stored in skeletal muscles, with the reminder found in the heart, brain and testes An average sized healthy male may have about 4 ounces (120 grams) of creatine stored in his body. When creatine is used during work or exercise, the body normally makes another 2 grams a day.

To increase sports performance, creatine is usually

taken in up to 5 gram doses, one to four times a day. To obtain 5 grams of creatine from steak would require about 2.4 pounds (1.1 kilograms). Vegetarians have little creatine in their diets.

THERAPEUTIC USES
- increases exercise tolerance
- increases muscular strength
- increases physical endurance

BEST FOOD SOURCES

Food	Creatine (mg/100g)
Beef	2.0
Cod	1.4
Herring	3.0
Salmon	2.0
Tuna	2.0
Milk	0.05
Cranberries	0.009

TOXICITY, CAUTIONS AND CONTRAINDICATIONS
No known toxicity or side effects.

DEHYDROEPIANDROSTERONE (DHEA)

DESCRIPTION

Scientists may never find a magic substance that can turn back the clock, but they are constantly hunting for clues for substances, which can make people feel more vigorous as they grow older. Researchers have found that administration of a male androgen hormone called dehydroepiandrosterone (DHEA) has remarkable effects in middle-aged and elderly subjects. Restoring DHEA levels to those of a typical 20-year-old person among subjects aged 40 to 70 years vastly improved the physical and psychological well being in both men and women.

These and other studies show that DHEA not only improved energy levels, but also increased muscle mass, mental acuity and immune function. Subjects noted a reversal in the increasing catabolism associated with aging and told researchers they felt more like they did in their twenties. No negative side effects were reported in these short-term studies, leading to speculation that DHEA may help people suffer fewer nagging aches and pains.

After about age 35, most people gradually lose muscle mass, become fatigued more easily, and find that their immune systems are not as good at fighting off diseases as when they were younger. Some of these changes are due to inactivity and lifestyle changes. However, even people who exercise a lot and watch their diet are nonetheless subject to the aging process. Muscle function deteriorates with age, in part because of a loss of muscle-building hormones, including DHEA. Of course, this has important implications to body builders.

DHEA is produced mainly in the adrenal glands, and to a lesser extent in the gonads. It is more highly concentrated in the bloodstream than any other steroid hormone made from cholesterol. It first appears in the bloodstream by the age of seven and reaches its peak at about age 25. After that, production declines gradually, so that by about age 60, it has decreased by almost 90 percent from peak levels. Hormones such as testosterone also decrease with age, but not to the same extent as DHEA. Scientists speculate that the large decrease in this hormone plays an important part in the aging process.

DHEA is linked to many important bodily functions. In addition to preserving muscle mass, it appears to play a role in strengthening the immune system, controlling body fat, and preventing depression.

As DHEA declines, several negative consequences occur. There is loss of muscle mass and stamina, fatigue, increase of body fat, decline in sex drive, and increased illness. Many of these negative effects diminish when people are given DHEA. In studies, administration of DHEA also improved feelings of well being.

THERAPEUTIC USES
- improves energy levels
- increases muscle mass
- improves mental acuity
- improves immune function
- reduces risk of bladder and other cancers
- inhibits carcinogenesis
- reduces the incidence of atherosclerosis

TOXICITY, CAUTIONS & CONTRAINDICATIONS:
Blood lavel must be monitored

DIMETHYL SULFONE (MSM)

DESCRIPTION

Sulfur plays an indispensable and unfortunately often overlooked role in human nutrition, responsible for maintaining the conformation of the body's proteins by forming flexible disulfide bonds between certain amino acids. It has a critical role in maintaining the integrity of connective tissue and the functions of many of the body's enzymes. To perform properly our bodies need a constant intake of easily available sulfur.

Dimethyl sulfone, also called MSM, is a naturally occurring form of organic sulfur found in all living organisms. It is present at a low concentration in human body fluids and tissue, as well as in many common foods, including milk, meat, fish, and a variety of fruits, vegetables and grains. However, when foods are processed, heated or dried, the essential MSM is lost. Therefore, unless a person's diet is composed primarily of raw foods, it is unlikely that he or she is receiving enough MSM for proper health. Research suggests that maintaining a minimum concentration in the body may be critical to normal functioning, and that the level of MSM in the body drops with increasing age. Good health practices involve replacing such declining essential substances, and the most effective and convenient way to prevent a sulfur-deficient diet is to replenish the body's MSM with a regular dietary supplement. MSM is an odorless, essentially tasteless, water-soluble, white, crystalline substance that serves as an important, bioavailable source of dietary sulfur.

When incorporated into a gel or lotion and applied to the skin, purified MSM softens, smoothes, soothes, and makes older skin more pliable. The results have been quite remarkable. Except for its beneficial inhibitory effect on cross-linking collagen and proteins, whereby it reduces hardening of skin and connective tissue, MSM appears to be inert in tissues and body fluids. Because of inertness, MSM is non-allergenic and non-pyretic, and has no interfering or undesirable pharmacological effects.

THERAPEUTIC USES

- protects against many allergens by competing for mucous membrane receptor sites
- combats environmental allergies such as house dust, pollen, wool, animal hair, and feathers
- alleviates allergic response to drugs, non-steroidal anti-inflammatory agents, oral antibiotics, and various foods
- relieves symptoms of pain and inflammation associated with injuries and physical stress
- alleviates arthritis pain
- ameliorates gastrointestinal upset
- active against Giardiai lamblia (traveler's diarrhea), Trichomonads and roundworms

TOXICITY, CAUTIONS & CONTRAINDICATIONS

MSM has exceedingly low toxicity to all forms of plant and animal life, exhibiting this low toxicity by any route of administration. Some have reported greater benefit when used in combination with vitamin C, especially for pain.

DOCOSAHEXAENOIC ACID (DHA)

DESCRIPTION

Docosahexaenoic acid (DHA, not to be confused with DHEA) is an omega-3 long-chain polyunsaturated fatty acid. It is important because it is the primary building block of the brain and retina of the eye. The brain is 60 percent fat. DHA is the primary structural fatty acid in the gray matter of the brain and retina of the eye. Thus it is essential for brain and eye function. It is also the most abundant fatty acid in human breast milk.

The human body synthesizes a small amount of DHA naturally, but the primary source is dietary, being found in eggs, red meats, fish, and animal organ meats. Many people avoid these foods because of the high concentration of "bad" saturated fats, but one result is a deficiency of DHA. Today, the average American's daily intake of DHA is estimated to be 100 mg lower than it was about 50 years ago. Similarly, the level of DHA in the breast milk of American women is significantly below what it was 50 years ago, and is one of the lowest in the world. An additional 200 mg of DHA per day returns the breast milk of the average American mother to near historical levels.

If a person eats at least one serving of fatty fish such as salmon or sea bass per day, he or she is likely getting enough DHA from dietary sources, but mercury and other contaminants are a concern, especially in pregnant or lactating women. Fish oil supplements can also supply abundant DHA (see the following section). Vegetarians, however, can take encouragement in the fact that DHA is now being extracted from microalgal sources.

FISH OILS

DESCRIPTION

Omega-3 is a name given to a group of essential fatty acids - called "essential" because the body cannot manufacture them and they must therefore come from the diet. They are derived primarily from oily fish, such as mackerel, salmon and herring.

The importance of omega-3 in fish oils was discovered when it was determined that the people of the Inuit tribe of Native Americans (Eskimos) have very low blood cholesterol levels despite a diet that includes the highest animal fat content of any diet in the world.

Omega-3 fatty acids have been found to reduce a group of fats called triglycerides. High levels of triglycerides impair the body's ability to break down blood clots, which contribute to the risk of heart attack, arrhythmias, and stroke. Fish oils have been found to reduce the viscosity of the blood, therefore facilitating blood flow. Omega-3 fatty acids can be obtained by consuming oily fish regularly. A 20-year study in The Netherlands (1960-1980), which involved middle-aged men without a history of coronary heart disease, demonstrated that those who consumed at least 1.1 oz. of fish a day had only half the mortality rate from heart attacks as those who ate no fish. In Bristol in 1983, a study was set up to determine whether men who had already suffered a heart attack could reduce the risk of further heart attacks by a change in their diet. The results demonstrated that men who had increased their consumption of fatty fish had 29 percent fewer deaths than the group that did not.

However, mercury and other contaminants in today's fish have made daily fish consumption problematic, especially in those pregnant or breastfeeding. Fortunately, the omega-3 fatty acids can also be obtained by supplementing with salmon oil, an excellent natural source of omega-3 fatty acids that can have most contaminants removed. Cod liver oil is another supplemental sources of omega-3 fatty acids. It also contains large amounts of vitamins A and D, making it a good choice especially in the autumn and winter months since less sun exposure will potentially result in less vitamin D production.

An important area of research is the link between essential fatty acids, birth weight and intelligence. Babies require both of the essential fatty acids, omega-3 (as in fish and flax seed oils) and omega-6 (as in most vegetable oils), for normal development.

THERAPEUTIC USES

- rheumatoid arthritis (shown to reduce the symptoms of swelling, tenderness, morning stiffness, and pain)
- eczema, acne and psoriasis

TOXICITY, CAUTIONS & CONTRAINDICATIONS

Fish oil has been used in very high amounts in clinical research without any overt toxicity symptoms. However, therapeutic levels of fish oil intake should be monitored by a medical professional, because omega-3 fatty acids can displace omega-6 fatty acids from cell membranes. There may also be a thinning of the blood and a resulting change in clotting time.

As mentioned above, excessive fish intake may cause accumulation of the toxic contaminants found in today's fish. This is especially important in pregnant or lactating women. Fish oils and evening primrose oil can suitably be supplemented together to achieve a balance of the two families of fatty acids (omega-3 and omega-6). However, ideal ratios between the two are still debated.

Occasionally, fish oil supplements may cause nausea when first taken. This symptom subsides over a period of

time and can be lessened by taking the dosage with a meal.
Those on blood-thinning drugs such as warfarin should avoid fish oils.

FLAXSEED OIL

DESCRIPTION

Organic flax seed oil is an important source of alpha-linolenic acid (ALA), an omega-3 series of essential fatty acids. ALA is the precursor to eicosapentaenoic acid and the Series 3 prostaglandins (PGE3), which are critical hormones regulating cellular activity.

The PGE 3 series prostaglandins, along with PGE 1 series prostaglandins, protect the body against the deleterious effects of PGE 2 series prostaglandins such as high blood pressure, sticky platelets, inflammation, water retention and lowered immune function. The series 2 prostaglandins are made from the omega-6 family of fatty acids and from consumption of excess animal products.

Numerous studies have shown that omega-3 fatty acids help lower cholesterol and blood triglycerides, and help prevent clots in arteries, which may result in strokes, heart attacks and thromboses.

Immunity is the body's ability to defend itself successfully against foreign substances. Flaxseed contains two components that may improve immune function: Alpha Linolenic Acid and Lignans. Recent research suggests that ALA and Lignans in Flaxseed modulet the immune response and may play a beneficial role in the clinical management of autoimmuno deseases. Flaxseed appears to protect against certain cancers in humans, particularly hormone-sensitive cancers such as those of the breast and endometrium and prostate.

Multiple studies have well documented the role of ALA in the prevention of artherosclerosis, which is the underline cause of many cardiovascular diseases including heart attack.

TOXICITY, CAUTIONS & CONTRAINDICATIONS:

Not known

GLUCOSAMINE SULFATE

DESCRIPTION

Glucosamine, an amino sugar normally formed in the body from glucose, is the starting point for the synthesis of many important macromolecules including glycoproteins, glycolipids, and glycos-aminoglycans (mucopolysaccharides). The tissues containing these glucosamine macromolecules include tendons and ligaments, cartilage, synovial fluid, mucous membranes, several structures in the eyes, blood vessels, and heart valves. A deficiency of glucosamine can reduce the rate of production of these important macromolecules, thereby leading to tissue weakness. In certain cases of trauma to these tissues, the amount of glucosamine normally synthesized by the body is insufficient.

Together with its associated macromolecules, glucosamine sulfate helps to make the synovial fluid thick and elastic in the joints, including those of the spine. Tissues in the joints can become damaged when the lubricating synovial fluids in the joint spaces become thin and watery. Normal cushioning is lost. Bones and their cartilage scrape against each other inside the joint space. Weakened bursal sacs around the joints can also cause tendons to rub against the hard edges of bones, increasing the possibility of inflammation and causing problems with movement and flexibility.

These problems can also occur in the spinal column where the individual vertebrae are stacked on top of each other, separated only by the cushioning intervertebral disc. The spaces between the vertebrae are where nerves leave the spinal cord, which increases the value of maintaining the height of these cushioning discs. Any injury to this area can cause the gelatinous cartilage to soften and thin. When this happens, pressure may be put directly upon the nerves. Glucosamine sulfate helps increase the thickness of the gelatinous material, creating more support for both the joints and vertebrae.

Glucosamine sulfate, which is naturally found in high concentrations in joint structures, appears to be one substance that can help with symptoms of osteoarthritis. Glucosamine sulfate has been shown to exert a protective effect against joint destruction and is selectively used by joint tissues, exerting a powerful healing effect on arthritic symptoms.

Glucosamine sulfate is not an analgesic or an anti-inflammatory agent; rather it appears to halt the disease process. Improvements occur more slowly with glucosamine sulfate than with over-the-counter arthritis medications, e.g., non-steroidal anti-inflammatory drugs (NSAIDs) such as ibuprofen. Eventually, however, glucosamine overtakes the NSAIDs in terms of effectiveness. Tests have shown that over time, glucosamine sulfate outperform NSAIDs and other traditional arthritis medications.

THERAPEUTIC USES

- combats breakdown and inflammation of synovial membranes
- helps repair damaged tissues such as ligaments and muscles
- relieves inflamed spinal discs
- relieves symptoms of osteoarthritis

GREEN–LIPPED MUSSEL

DESCRIPTION

Laboratory-based investigations of a commercially prepared freeze-dried extract of the green-lipped mussel (Perna canaliculus) showed that the material had the capacity to inhibit experimentally induced inflammation. The activity was thought to reside within an aqueous fraction containing high molecular weight material, possibly a polysaccharide.

In one study, a polysaccharide (glycogen) was extracted from Perna canaliculus and its anti-inflammatory activity was examined. The high molecular weight material was administered I.V. and demonstrated a dose-dependent anti-inflammatory effect in rats with carrageenan-induced footpad edema. Mobilization of neutrophils to the site of the inflammatory stimulus was significantly reduced. This activity was lost if the glycogen extract was treated with KOH or proteinase K, suggesting that the anti-inflammatory properties reside within a protein molecule associated with the glycogen.

TOXICITY, CAUTIONS & CONTRAINDICATIONS

Not known

GLUTATHIONE

DESCRIPTION

Glutathione is a natural, sulfur-containing peptide (very small protein). The roles of glutathione in the body are numerous and varied. Historically, most of the research interest has been in the role of glutathione in amino acid transport across cell membranes. Recently, biochemists have been excited by glutathione's role as an antioxidant, detoxifier, and the possible reversal of malignant cells to healthy cells. Glutathione is formed by linking three amino acids together; glutamic acid, cysteine and glycine. Glutathione is highly soluble in water and largely absorbed intact with approximately 80 percent of an oral dose reaching the bloodstream within three hours.

Glutathione, cysteine, and certain sulfur-containing proteins form an important "pool" of compounds that are responsible for maintaining the proper oxidation state in the body. They return certain oxidized compounds back to their normal forms. Glutathione itself is an important water-soluble antioxidant and free-radical scavenger. Glutathione is a key antioxidant factor, but there still is much more to the glutathione-antioxidant story. Glutathione teams with a selenium-containing enzyme called glutathione peroxidase, which directly deactivates free radicals, especially of the lipid peroxide type. This important enzyme does not function in the absence of glutathione.

GLUTATHIONE AND AGING RESEARCH

Glutathione's synergism with the antioxidant nutrients vitamin E and selenium attracted experimental interest in aging research. It is interesting to note that glutathione levels of aged cells are 20-30 percent lower than young cells. Research efforts are underway to attempt to discover if there is a cause and effect relationship. Glutathione has many roles and in none does it act alone. It is coenzyme in various enzymatic reactions. Glutathione (especially in the liver) binds with toxic chemicals in order to detoxify them. We are likely to be exposed to many of the pollutants glutathione detoxifies: radiation, pesticides, herbicides, fungicides, plastics, nitrates, cigarette smoke, and birth control pills. Glutathione also detoxifies heavy metals such as lead, cadmium, and mercury. In addition to glutathione's direct chemical detoxifying reactions and its indirect detoxifying reactions teamed with glutathione peroxidase, it also improves the immune system's ability to destroy bacteria and remove "debris". It is also important in red and white blood cell formation and throughout the immune system. Special white blood cells called phagocytes have improved function and are less subject to chemical inhibition when well-nourished with glutathione.

GLUTATHIONE AND CANCER

The detoxifying properties of glutathione, especially its ability to destroy highly carcinogenic epoxides and peroxides, has drawn early attention by those experimenting with cancer protection. But recent research is examining the possibility that glutathione may destroy liver cancer. An article was published in Science in 1981 that indicated glutathione destroyed aflatoxin-induced liver cancer in laboratory rats. Other scientists are now duplicating this research for confirmation. As Dr. A. Novi, a German scientist reported in Science, "the effect of glutathione, a harmless natural product, on (induced liver cancer) in rats strongly suggests that this antioxidant merits further investigation as a potential antitumor agent in humans."

GLUTATHIONE, NITRIC OXIDE AND CIRCULATION

"Glutathione peroxidase increases the inhibitor effect of nitric oxide on platelet aggregation by reducing hydroperoxides. Moreover, other authors have shown that glutathion favorably influences the coronary circluation. In fact, the intracoronary infusion of reduced glutathione improves endothelial vasomotor response in subjects with coronary risk factors and nitroglycerin.

GLUTATHIONE EFFECTS LIVER AND BRAIN DETOXIFICATION

Glutathione is one of the most important components of the liver's detoxification system. Of special interest is the liver protection provided by glutathione against alcohol. While the ability to detoxify various chemicals to which we are exposed is different for each individual, those, whose detoxification pathways are blocked are at far greater risk to the brain damaging effects of a wide variety of toxins. Giving glutathione is one of the most effective techniques for enhancing liver and brain detoxification. The concept of enhancing cellular receptor sensitivity has become quite familiar in medicine today. Glutathione has the unique ability to make certain areas of the brain more sensitive to the neurotransmitter, called dopamine. Increasing glutathione levels decreases free radical and mitochondrial damage, which can lead to neuronal degeneration. Glutathione is a critically important brain chemical. It is clearly one of the most important brain antioxidants, that is, glutathione helps to preserve brain tissue by preventing damage from free radicals – destructive chemicals formed by the normal processes of metabolism, toxic elements in the environment and as a normal response of the body to challenges by infectious agents and other stresses. In addition to quenching dangerous free radicals, glutathione also acts to recycle vitamin C and vitamin E, which because of their antioxidant activity, also reduce free radicals in the brain.

TOXICITY:
Not known

HISTIDINE–RICH GLYCOPROTEIN

DESCRIPTION

Histidine is an amino acid that is essential for the growth and repair of tissues. Histidine-rich glycoprotein (HRG) is a relatively abundant plasma glycoprotein in humans, whose function is still a matter of debate. It contains about 15% carbohydrate and an unusually high proportion of histidine and proline, hence the name histidine-proline-rich glycoprotein would better reflect the amino acid composition.

The precise physiological role of HRG is not known, although several functions have been proposed based on its binding abilities. Histidine is intricately involved in a large number of critical metabolic processes, ranging from the production of red and white blood cells to regulating antibody activity. It also helps to maintain the myelin sheaths, which surround and insulate nerves. In particular, histidine has been found beneficial for the auditory nerves, and a deficiency of this vital amino acid has been noted in cases of nerve deafness. Histidine is required for the production of histamine, and is often used in the treatment of anemia, allergies, rheumatoid arthritis and other inflammatory reactions.

Histidine also possesses vasodilating and hypotensive actions and may have an important role in sexual responses. Women who are unable to achieve orgasm may be low in histamine and can possibly benefit from histidine. Histidine seems to boost the activity of suppressor T cells. Research has shown abnormally low levels of histidine in the blood of patients with rheumatoid arthritis. It is also used as a chelating agent in some cases of arthritis and to treat tissue overload from copper, iron and other heavy metals to help remove them from the body. It acts as an inhibitory neurotransmitter, boosting the activity of alpha waves in the brain and supporting resistantance to the effects of anxiety and stress. In case of histidine deficiency, there is an unbalancing effect on alpha rhythms, leading to greater beta wave production. It is naturally found in most animal and vegetable proteins, particularly in poultry, cheese, and wheat germ.

Histidine must be obtained from diet during childhood and growth periods. It is necessary in malnourished or injured individuals, or whenever there is need for tissue formation or repair.

Typical daily therapeutic doses range from 1000 mg to 1500 mg.

THERAPEUTIC USES
- arthritis
- anemia
- sexual dysfunction in women

TOXICITY, CAUTIONS & CONTRAINDICATIONS
Not known

HUMAN GROWTH HORMONE

DESCRIPTION

Human growth hormone (somatotropin) is a water-soluble protein with a short half-life in blood (20 minutes). It is a general growth-controlling hormone, which controls insulin. It is also one of the least understood hormones, its mode of action remaining unclear. The chief functions of human growth hormone are to stimulate protein, fat, carbohydrate, water, and mineral metabolism, as well as to enhance general body growth. Its importance stems from its role as a central hormone in the pituitary as well as its control of body metabolism in the tissues via synergism and antagonism with the other pituitary hormones.

Of the many hormones produced by the endocrine glands, somatotropin is one of the most abundant. Its production by the pituitary gland begins to decline during the teenage years and continues to decline throughout adulthood at the rate of about 14 percent per decade. Toward the end of a typical life span, production has dropped to a small fraction of that of a young person.

Supplemental human growth hormone is one of the most controversial topics in health today. There is no doubt that it has helped many young people with hypopituitarism (dwarfism) to reach a normal human height and proportion. More recently, it has been used by adults who claim significant help in combating the effects of chronic diseases that involve wasting, such as stroke, chronic obstructive pulmonary disease, and AIDS.

Human growth hormone also appears to help regulate body fat. After six months of HGH treatment at Sahlgrenska Hospital in Sweden, somatotropin-deficient adults lost 20 percent of their body fat. Most of this fat loss occurred in abdominal fat, which was reduced by 30 percent compared with a 13 percent reduction in peripheral fat, in the arms and legs. It is abdominal fat that is strongly correlated with increased risk of heart attack, hypertension, and diabetes.

Growth hormone is normally released by GHRH, a hypothalamic releasing factor, or by sleep, exercise, fasting, hypoglycemia, or the amino acid, arginine. Release-inhibiting factors include GH-RIH (somatostatin), sleeplessness, hyperglycemia, obesity, and free fatty acids. Because growth hormone controls the nitrogen balance of an organism, it is thought to be involved in the aging process. In a study published in The New England Journal of Medicine, July 5th, 1990, Daniel Rudman, M.D., states, "Six months of HGH therapy reversed the aging process from 10 to 20 years!" Nonetheless, adverse long-term effects are still a concern.

THERAPEUTIC USES
- dwarfism (hypopituitarism)
- possibly to reduce fat and build muscle

TOXICITY, CAUTIONS & CONTRAINDICATIONS
Toxicity has been reported. The diabetogenic and carcinogenic effect is well known. Excess somatotropin results in acromegaly and gigantism. Its chief synergists are insulin, testosterone, Mg^{2+}, Zn^{2+}, and K^+, whereas its chief antagonist is cortisol. Opponents of growth hormone use claim many negative side effects.

5–HYDROXYTRYPTOPHAN (5–HTP)

DESCRIPTION

Researchers have discovered that many of us suffer from a little-known deficiency of serotonin in brain tissue. An important neurotransmitter, serotonin regulates key functions related to mood, sleep, and appetite. Deficiencies can result in mild to severe depression, weight problems, and migraine headaches.

Prescription drugs such as Prozac, which increases availability of serotonin in the brain, have been developed to treat depression. However, side effects of Prozac and other selective serotonin reuptake inhibitors (SSRI's) can be significant. Researchers have been conducting studies, which show that you can increase serotonin availability by taking supplements of the metabolic precursors of serotonin, the amino acids tryptophan or 5-hydroxytryptophan (5-HTP). Unfortunately, tryptophan was removed from the market as a supplement. However, 5-HTP, which is the next precursor on the metabolic pathway to serotonin, is available for use as a supplement and has actually proven to be superior to tryptophan in clinical trials, potentially providing a safer alternative to drugs such as Prozac.

When double blind clinical trials compared tryptophan to 5-HTP in treating depression, the 5-HTP was found to be clearly superior. Other studies conducted by a team of Swiss and German psychiatric researchers headed by Dr. W. Poldinger of the Psychiatric University of Basel, Switzerland showed a nearly equal reduction in treating depression with 5-HTP as compared to the anti-depressant drug, fluvoxamine. 5-HTP also appeared to be better tolerated.

Other studies have shown significant reductions in anxiety with 5-HTP. In a study of 20 people with panic disorders, several experienced relief after taking 5-HTP.

5-HTP has been used to treat depression and anxiety. One of serotonin's metabolic pathways leads directly to the production of melatonin, a sleep-enhancing hormone. 5-HTP, as a serotonin precursor, has therefore been used to relieve insomnia.

5-HTP has also been used to treat obesity and migraine headaches. An Italian study conducted on 20 obese patients showed that the patients taking larger doses of 5-HTP experienced a significant weight loss, had less carbohydrate intake and consistently ate less than the placebo group. The study concluded that 5-HTP was well tolerated and could be safely used as an obesity treatment. A Spanish study showed 71 percent improvement in migraine sufferers, while Italian researchers confirmed a 90 percent improvement in headache severity, frequency and duration with 400 mg/day of 5-HTP for a period of 2 months.

THERAPEUTIC USES
- depression
- anxiety and insomnia
- obesity
- migraine headaches

KELP

DESCRIPTION

Known as "seaweed" or "brown algae," kelp has a number of therapeutic properties. A regular food in the Japanese diet, it helps to regulate the metabolism. It provides nourishment for proper functioning of the thyroid in the form of organic iodine, and strengthens tissues in the heart and brain. It contains approximately 30 trace and major minerals vital to health, including high levels of natural calcium, potassium and magnesium (excellent for nails, hair and skin). It also supports the elimination of waste and toxic metals from the body. Kelp enhances health and can help rebuild the immune system. This relative of blue-green algae has a component called "fucoidan" which has demonstrated exciting medicinal potential. In animal studies, fucoidan has been shown to have anticoagulant and fibrinolytic activities.

Seaweeds such as nori (the paper-thin one which is used to wrap certain kinds of sushi), wakame (the one which is boiled and used as an ingredient in Japanese miso soup), and some other edible varieties contain sodium alginate, which has been shown to remove free radical-producing heavy metals and radioactive isotopes from the body. With the use of kelp, the thyroid is amply supplied with iodine, and it will not absorb more. Therefore, if one is exposed to radioactive iodine, it will just pass through the body. One famous example of this is the story of the people in the hospital in Hiroshima who survived the atomic bomb blast although people in their vicinity died from radiation sickness. They had been on a strict macrobiotic diet, which included lots of seaweed. There is some suggestion that brown algae helps ward off cancer and that it is the copious amounts of nori in the Japanese diet that accounts for the exceptionally low rate of breast cancer in that country.

There are two ways to add this important ingredient to your nutritional regimen and using both methods is recommended. One is to obtain kelp supplements from your health food store and take them daily. The other is to use nori, wakame, and other seaweed products in your diet. These are readily obtainable from Asian food sections of markets. If you go out for sushi, ask for nori-maki, the kind that is wrapped in seaweed.

On a cautionary note, there is a Japanese kelp variety known as "kombu" which is the organic source of monosodium glutamate, or MSG. Some packaged food producers list "seaweed" as an ingredient when what they actually have added is MSG. Consider the source.

KOMBUCHA

DESCRIPTION

The ancient, yeast-culture "panacea," kombucha, also known as "Manchurian mushroom ," takes seven days to reproduce itself. It looks like a six-inch-diameter pancake but is grayish in color. As a tea, it contains a concentrated amount of high quality protein, which the body digests and uses immediately. Yeast enzymes respond to the living microorganisms in the body, where they are metabolized readily.

The first recorded use of kombucha tea was during the Chinese empire of the Tsin Dynasty in 221 B.C. In 414 B.C. Dr. Kombu, from Korea, brought it to Japan. Afterwards, this tea was used throughout China, Japan and Korea and later introduced to Russia and India.

The Kombucha fungus is built in membrane form and is a symbiosis of yeast cells and different bacteria. Among these bacteria are: Bacterium xylinum, B. gluconicum, Acetobacter ketogenum and Pichia fermentans.

The kombucha fungi need to live in a solution composed of black tea and sugar. In the right temperature they multiply constantly in a process which produces glucuronic acid, lactic acid, acetic acid and several vitamins. The yeast culture transforms the sugar and black tea into enzymes useful for the body.

Commonly sold as a bottled beverage in ordinary grocery stores in Europe, the fermented mixture contains 0.5 percent alcohol, glucuronic acid, which is used in the body to build important polysacharides such as hyaluronic acid, which is vital for the connective tissues; chondroitin sulfate, which is the basic building block of cartilage; mukoitin sulfate, which is necessary for mucus and for the vitreous humor of the eye; and lactic acid, which especially benefits the colon.

THERAPEUTIC USES

- natural antibiotic, as in infectious diarrhea.
- enhances blood circulation and the metabolism
- liver and kidney disorders
- indigestion, in part by supporting the intestinal flora
- bronchitis, asthma, and coughs
- weight reduction
- high uric acid (gout) or cholesterol
- rheumatism and arthritis
- muscular aches and pains
- allergies
- may help eliminate cataracts and other formations on the cornea
- hypertension
- boils and skin diseases (eliminates wrinkles and helps remove brown spots)
- helps level off blood glucose levels, especially in diabetics
- thickens hair
- reduces hot flashes during menopause
- stress reduction

Just after drinking the Manchurian mushroom tea, one may feel a warm sensation due to the fact that the tea components join the blood stream causing a "draining" action of toxic chemical elements and fluids. For this reason, one may notice increased mobility in the extremities and flexibility around the waist.

L-CARNITINE

DESCRIPTION

L-Carnitine was first discovered several decades ago, but only recently have researchers found that it actually stimulates the rate of fat burning. This observation prompted extensive clinical research into the potential applications of L-Carnitine so that today, thanks to mounting scientific evidence, it is widely accepted that L-Carnitine plays a crucial role in cardiovascular metabolism, exercise performance, weight management, infant nutrition and optimal brain function.

L-Carnitine is an amino acid-like and vitamin B-like substance, which can exist in two forms, the D- and L-isomers (isomers are compounds which have same the chemical make up but are mirror images of each other, similar to one's left and right hands). Only the L-isomer, L-Carnitine, is found in nature and is biologically active. In fact, the D form is biologically inactive and because of its potential negative effects, the sale of D-Carnitine and D, L-Carnitine (a mixture of the two isomeric forms) is banned in the U.S.

Dietary sources of L-Carnitine consist primarily of foods of animal origin, particularly red meat (this obviously has important implications for vegetarians). Dietary L-Carnitine is absorbed in the small intestine. Endogenous synthesis in the body requires six other nutrients, including amino acids, vitamins and iron. Synthesis takes place primarily in the liver and kidney. Skeletal and heart muscle, which depend upon fat breakdown for energy, are highly dependent on L-Carnitine.

L-Carnitine plays a crucial role in fat breakdown and energy production. Basically, fat consists of three fatty acids linked to an alcohol molecule. The production of energy from fat requires that the fatty acids be transported from the cytosol of the cell into the mitochondria for beta oxidation, or "fat burning." Although fatty acids by themselves are unable to penetrate the inner mitochondrial membrane, a transport system consisting of L-Carnitine and at least three enzymes shuttles the long chain fatty acids into the mitochondria. Thus, one of the most fundamental roles of L-Carnitine is in the transport of long chain fatty acids across the mitochondrial membrane. Inside the cell's powerhouse, mitochondria, the fatty acids are broken down and energy is ultimately produced. Therefore, L-Carnitine is essential for fat metabolism and energy production.

The secondary function of L-Carnitine is to shuttle short chain fatty acids from inside the mitochondria to the cytosol. This detoxification action of L-Carnitine is of significance because it allows fat burning and energy production to continue inside the mitochondria.

LECITHIN

DESCRIPTION

Lecithin, from the Greek word for egg yolk, "lekithos," is a fat emulsifier. It is made by the liver but is also found in egg yolk. It was first isolated in 1850. Lecithin is a "natural emulsifier," important in emulsification of fats. It is rich in B-vitamin factors and phosphorus. It breaks down body fat so that the fat may be transported to the liver and converted into a usable energy food.

Lecithin and cholesterol are necessary for the renewal and maintenance of all cell membranes. The sheaths surrounding the nerves in our bodies contain lecithin and the brain requires lecithin to function properly. A complex mixture of fats and essential fatty acids, lecithin itself is predominantly fat, combined with phosphorus and choline.

Lecithin in the diet does not necessarily increase the lecithin in the blood. As lecithin is digested, the molecules are broken down and then pass through the intestinal walls to become, as needed, part of the lipoprotein complex, which performs the necessary function of transporting cholesterol through the blood. When the B-complex vitamins and in particular vitamin B6 are present, the body will manufacture its own lecithin. A common ingredient found in many food products, lecithin has the ability to combine oil with water-based ingredients. However, lecithin has earned itself a reputation as a vital factor in the prevention and treatment of heart disease, and as a positive slimming aid. Lecithin plays a part in the prevention of pulmonary edema. It is also essential in preventing certain types of arteriosclerosis (hardening of the arteries) by allowing cholesterol to pass through artery walls.

Lecithin has unusual therapeutic properties and many variable functions. It is a natural substance capable of dispersing fat globules into smaller units (necessary for proper emulsification) without the aid of artificial emulsifying agents. By ingesting lecithin, we can get its B-vitamin factors (choline and inositol), and its other vital components, particularly the mineral phosphorus and unsaturated fatty acids.

Medical science is fascinated by lecithin, with its cellular omnipresence and its therapeutic properties. Lecithin helps food retain moisture, and combats nutrient loss by retarding oxidation. Research indicates it has the capacity to aid in the absorption of vitamin A. Researchers also have found lecithin forms 30 percent of a healthy human brain's dry weight, and over 70 percent of the liver's substance.

Research has shown that atherosclerosis can be reversed via reduction of blood cholesterol and lipids to normal levels. Pure soybean lecithin, when regularly incorporated into the diet, lowers cholesterol. Lecithin and cholesterol co-exist in equilibrium, with lecithin controlling cholesterol.

As an emulsifier, lecithin breaks down fat. Large particles of fat act as a platform upon which sticky platelets collect, that can go on to reduce blood circulation and eventually lead to blood clots. Various studies on those with coronary heart disease have shown low levels of blood lecithin, with a corresponding increased risk of blood clotting.

Soy lecithin keeps fat from forming deposits, breaking it up into small particles, which can be metabolized more easily and thoroughly than larger particles.

THERAPEUTIC USES

- helps liver bile emulsify fats and cholesterol
- helps to normalize low phospholipid-to-cholesterol ratios found in patients with gallstones (minimum dose of 2g per day)
- may benefit a small number of patients with

advanced Alzheimer's disease, improving orientation, learning, and memory (controversial)

- lecithin or choline supplements may help slow the deterioration of nerve coverings (some evidence that lecithin content of myelin is depleted in multiple sclerosis)

TOXICITY, CAUTIONS & CONTRAINDICATIONS

Lecithin does not have any reported side effects at levels up to 100g per day for up to four months. In Alzheimer's patients taking drugs for this condition, lecithin may cause gastrointestinal disturbances.

LUTEIN

DESCRIPTION

Lutein is found in certain fruits and vegetables as well as egg yolks. It is a nutrient with a number of potentially beneficial effects. It is a member of the carotenoid family, a group of chemicals related to vitamin A . While beta-carotene, the precursor of vitamin A, may be the most familiar carotenoid, there are almost 600 others whose effects have yet to be extensively studied. Aside from lutein, these include alpha-carotene, lycopene, zeaxanthin, and beta-cryptoxanthin. In the plant world, carotenoids like lutein help to give color to sweet potatoes, carrots, and other fruits and vegetables. In people, lutein and zeaxanthin make up most of the pigment in the center of the retina, where vision sensitivity is greatest. While lutein is not considered an essential nutrient, studies suggest that it may play an important role in maintaining healthy vision and preventing eye diseases such as age-related macular degeneration (ARMD) and cataracts. Getting adequate amounts of this carotenoid may also decrease the risk of developing colon cancer and heart disease .

Lutein and other carotenoids are considered important because of their antioxidant properties. Antioxidants help to protect cells from damage caused by free radicals, the destructive fragments of oxygen produced as a byproduct during normal metabolic processes. As free radicals travel through the body, they cause damage to cells and genes by stealing electrons from other molecules—a process referred to as oxidation. Test tube studies conducted by the Agricultural Research Service of the United States Department of Agriculture (USDA) suggest that lutein may be just as effective at combating free radicals as vitamin E , which is a potent antioxidant. Concentrated mainly in the lens and retina of the eye, lutein may help to protect vision by neutralizing free radicals and by increasing the density of eye pigment. Lutein may also shield the eyes from the destructive effects of sunlight. In one very small study, published in the journal Experimental Eye Research in 1997, lutein significantly reduced the amount of potentially damaging blue light that reached sensitive tissues in the eye. The study involved two people who received the equivalent of 30 mg of lutein a day for almost five months.

THERAPEUTIC USES

While not approved as a dietary supplement by the FDA, lutein is ubiquitous in foods. It may play an important role in maintaining vision and preventing such eye diseases as ARMD and cataracts, the two leading causes of vision loss in adults. The carotenoid may accomplish this by protecting eye tissue from free radical damage and shielding the eyes from potentially destructive sunlight. Research also indicates that getting adequate amounts of lutein may decrease the risk of colon cancer and heart disease. Lutein may offer protection against the latter two diseases by acting as an antioxidant, since free radical damage is believed to contribute to the development of cardiovascular disease as well as certain cancers.

Several studies with human subjects suggest that eating a diet high in lutein may help to keep the eyes healthy and prevent the development of ARMD and cataracts. It is important, however, to remember that fruits and vegetables containing lutein also contain a number of other nutrients. It is not known for certain if lutein is primarily responsible for protecting the eyes or if other nutrients in these foods are involved. The interaction of various nutrients may also play a therapeutic role. In one of these studies, published in the Journal of the American Medical Association in 1994, researchers examined the eating habits of almost 900 older adults. The goal was to investigate the relationship between ARMD and the intake of carotenoids as well as vitamins A, C, and E. Several hundred of the participants already had ARMD, while those in the control group were free of the disease. The results showed that those who had consumed the highest amount of carotenoids had a 43% lower risk for ARMD compared with those who ate the least amount. The researchers determined that lutein and zeaxanthin were primarily responsible for reducing the risk of ARMD. In terms of specific foods, spinach and collard greens (both rich in lutein) appeared to offer the most protection.

Lutein may also help to prevent the development of colon cancer, according to a study published in the American Journal of Clinical Nutrition in 2000. This study examined the risk of colon cancer and dietary intake of lutein and other carotenoids such as alpha-carotene, beta-carotene, lycopene, zeaxanthin, and beta-cryptoxanthin. The researchers examined the eating habits of over 4,000 people. Roughly half the participants were between the ages of 30 and 79 and already had colon cancer, while the remainder made up the cancer-free control group. The results indicated that men and women who had consumed large amounts of lutein were less likely to develop the disease. Interestingly, lutein was the only carotenoid identified by the study that seemed to offer any protection.

The evidence regarding lutein and heart disease is indirect but intriguing. In a four-week animal study conducted by researchers from the University of Southern California and the University of California at Los Angeles, some of the rodents were fed a diet rich in lutein while others received none. Due to a missing gene, the mice involved in the study were prone to develop rapid atherosclerosis. When the mice were killed and dissected, it was discovered that those on the lutein diet had much less plaque buildup in their arteries than those who did not receive the carotenoid. The study, which was presented at a meeting of the Federation of American Societies for Experimental Biology in 1999, suggests that lutein may offer protection against cardiovascular disease by preventing hardening of the arteries.

TOXICITY
Not known

LYCOPENE

DESCRIPTION

Lycopene is the red-colored carotenoid predominantly found in tomato fruit, but in few other fruits or vegetables. Lycopene is one of the most potent antioxidants among dietary carotenoids. Humans cannot synthesize carotenoids and have to depend upon the diet exclusively for the source of these micronutrients.

INGREDIENTS/USAGE

Dietary intake of tomatoes and tomato products containing Lycopene has been shown to be associated with a decreased risk of chronic diseases, such as cancer and cardiovascular disease.

The need of antioxidants is increased by the excess dietary fats, cigarette smoke, alcohol consumption, pollutants and stress.

A recent clinical study demonstrated that lycopene might not only prevent prostate cancer but also have therapeutic effects. Researchers in Finland have found that low plasma Lycopene concentrations are associated with early atherosclerosis, manifested as increased CCA-IMT (intima-media thickness of the common carotid artery wall), in middle-aged men living in eastern Finland.

A daily dose of Lycopene exerts a protective effect against EIA (exercise-induced asthma) in some patients, most probably through an in vivo antioxidative effect.

TOXICITY:

Not known

MAITAKE MUSHROOM

DESCRIPTION

The maitake mushroom, Grifola frondosa, is a polypore with pores under the cap instead of gills. It is a bracket fungus that grows on the trunks or stumps of trees or on the ground around them. Maitake (pronounced "my-tah-kee") is indigenous to northern Japan. For hundreds of years, this rare and tasty mushroom has been prized in traditional Japanese herbology. Maitake literally means "dancing mushroom." People who found the mushroom in deep mountains starting dancing with joy since they knew its delicious taste and the health benefits. Also, in the feudal era, it could be exchanged for the same weight of silver. Maitake was, and still is, one of the most valuable and expensive mushrooms in Japan. This is why this basketball-sized giant is called the "King of Mushrooms."

Mr. Shozo Goto, a master of mushroom hunting, stated in his book, "Mushroom Climate in Akita Prefecture" (1965), "Mushroom hunters have their own target mushrooms and hunting grounds. Top rank hunters are those who seek maitake. They go out to their own secret grounds to spend several days looking for maitake with a dream of fortune at a stroke. Maitake hunters are not supposed to let others know their secret spot. If one finds a spot where he can crop more than 10kg (22 lbs.) of maitake, he has found a 'Treasure Island.' He would never tell anyone his secret location until he dies, at which time he would only indicate the location in his will to his eldest son. Some hunters are even willing to die without telling their own sons or families..."

The legendary mushroom has been available by cultivation since the mid 1980's, which gave opportunities for mycologists and pharmacologists to study the various medicinal properties of maitake as claimed in anecdotes and folklore. In addition to its anti-tumor effects, antihypertensive and antidiabetic properties have been found in maitake. Its anti-HIV activity was also confirmed by the U.S. National Cancer Institute in early 1991.

The proteins in maitake mushrooms contain all of the essential amino acids and most commonly occurring non-essential amino acids and amides. Maitake are rich in vitamins, minerals, and fatty acids that are largely unsaturated. Key therapeutic substances are glucans, a major constituent of the cell walls. G. frondosa yields neutral D-glucans and acidic glucans.

THERAPEUTIC USES
- helps in reducing the risk of cancer
- lowers high blood pressure and cholesterol
- improves general immune response support

TOXICITY, CAUTIONS & CONTRAINDICATIONS
None noted. G. frondosa is edible when young.

MELATONIN

DESCRIPTION

Melatonin is the principle hormone produced and secreted by the pineal gland. The pineal gland through its secretion of melatonin is responsible for maintaining the body's circadian rhythm (biological clock) and regulating the endocrine (hormonal) system. The level of secretion of melatonin by the pineal gland is stimulated by the absence of sunlight. Inadequate melatonin secretion can cause disruptions in the sleep/wake cycle, headache, mental and physical fatigue, and irritability.

"Jet lag," the malaise that may occur after crossing more than two time zones in an airplane, can also be caused by working rotating shifts or by other disruptions of the normal sleep/wake cycle. Some people with "seasonal affective disorder" (SAD) experience this syndrome at times of the year (e.g. winter in northern areas) when levels of sunlight are insufficient to decrease melatonin production to normally low daytime levels. Melatonin supplementation can benefit these disturbances.

People without sleep disorders should take melatonin approximately one hour before going to bed. People with insomnia may wish to take melatonin two to three hours before the time they wish to fall asleep. For people wanting to fall asleep earlier than they currently do (including people trying to avoid jet lag), a melatonin supplement should be taken two to three hours before their new desired bedtime. The appropriate dosage can vary significantly from one person to another. For people under age 40 without sleep disorders and not wanting to change their circadian rhythm, it is prudent to start with a small dose such as 1 mg at the appropriate time. People over 40 who wish to change their circadian rhythm may want to start with 3 mg. If the person has slept well but is drowsy in the morning, then the dose can be cut in half. If the dose had little or no sleep-inducing effect, then the dose can be increased by 1 to 3 mg until the desired effect is achieved.

TOXICITY, CAUTIONS & CONTRAINDICATIONS

In supplement form, melatonin is considered to be nontoxic. However, melatonin supplements should not be taken by adolescents, pregnant or lactating women, people taking cortisone, or people with kidney disease.

PALM OIL

DESCRIPTION

Antioxidants, free radicals, and singlet oxygen species have been researched for decades. However, not until the recent past have the health implications of oxidative stress, the burden of a biological system to constantly try to neutralize and control the damaging effects of free radicals, come into their own. Internally generated cellular antioxidant systems are constantly operating, however, sufficient daily outside sources of antioxidants are also needed.

Carotenoids, including beta carotene, have significant yet differing functional and effective levels of biological activity, especially with respect to their role as antioxidants. Carrots are very comparable to palm oil in optimal carotenoid balance, whereas algae-derived carotenoids, although very rich in beta carotene, are less well balanced. Both crude palm oil and carrots are very rich in alpha carotene (30 to 50 percent) while algae (dunaliella) carotene runs about six to 10 percent. In many research studies, alpha carotene, although having about half the provitamin A activity of beta carotene, has about 10 times the power of beta carotene to inhibit skin, lung, and liver carcinogenesis.

Crude palm oil has other essential carotenoids. One of the most important carotenoids is lycopene. Although it does not have any provitamin A activity, lycopene is the most efficient biological singlet oxygen quencher of the carotenoids yet discovered. Lycopene has a quenching efficiency more than two times greater than beta carotene and 100 times greater than vitamin E.

While it appears that beta carotene is a very important plasma carotenoid, increased attention should be directed to other carotenoids such as lycopene, which actually has a higher plasma concentration than beta carotenoids. Lycopene has also been identified in low-density lipoproteins and therefore may function in the prevention of oxidation of LDL, causing atherosclerosis.

Physiological functions of other carotenoids found in crude palm oil may be highly specialized, as indicated by the presence of zeanthin and its isomer lutein in the macular area of the retina, while beta carotene is virtually absent. It is worthy to note that dark green vegetables are very high in lutein carotenoids. It is also important to note that crude palm oil carotenoid extract is devoid of any saturated fats, which are normally found in tropical oils.

The potential of crude palm oil carotenoid extract as an economical source of richly diversified carotenoids is enormous.

PHOSPHATIDYLSERINE (PS)

DESCRIPTION

Phosphatidylserine (PS) is a phospholipid that is vital to brain cell structure and function. Phospholipids are molecules with an amino acid "head" (serine for PS), and one or two fatty acid (lipid) "tails." They are found in the membranes of every cell in our bodies. The outer membrane of cells, including brain cells, is composed of a double layer of phospholipids, including PS, with their heads facing out and their tails facing inward toward each other. This double layer is responsible for bringing in nutrients, expelling wastes, and enabling the cell to coordinate with the rest of the body. The various proteins found in outer cell membranes, such as ion pumps, transport molecules, enzymes, antigens and receptors, are held in place and managed within the double layer. PS plays an important part in these functions, and the depletion of PS with age appears to be correlated with their decline.

PS is important for nerve cell activation (depolarization) and renewal (repolarization), and neurotransmitter production and release, thus maintaining electrical current flows in and between the cells.

According to the American Psychiatric Association, millions of healthy adults over age 50 are affected by "Age-Related Cognitive Decline," which results in diminished memory. At least 23 peer-reviewed studies, more than half of which were double-blinded, suggest that PS may help maintain or improve cognitive functions such as memory and learning in mature adults. The results in these well-controlled, published studies on PS, many of which involved individuals suffering from cognitive decline, included statistically significant improvements in measures of brain functions such as learning and remembering names of persons, recognizing people one has seen previously, remembering numeric information and the location of frequently misplaced objects, and improved concentration. Such results tend to substantiate the benefits of PS in relation to learning and memory. Although these and other results are encouraging, more studies are needed to complete our full understanding of the role of PS in brain function and to confirm that PS, when consumed as a dietary supplement, will consistently improve cognitive ability.

THERAPEUTIC USES

- memory, learning, and concentration
- people over 50 years of age and those who may have prematurely damaged brain cell membranes due to disease, alcohol, drug use, pollution, or other causes
- epilepsy (in support of conventional treatments)
- protection against stress hormone release, a negative adaptation to stress, which may occur in adults of any age

TOXICITY, CAUTIONS & CONTRAINDICATIONS

PS has been shown to be safe and effective for human use. Two hundred milligrams or more of PS taken at once may (rarely) cause nausea. Three hundred mg per day is associated with lower uric acid and liver SGPT levels, without adverse clinical effects. Because no reproductive studies appear to be available, most health care practitioners do not recommend PS for use in pregnant or nursing women.

PROANTHOCYANIDINS (PINE BARK EXTRACT)

DESCRIPTION

Pine bark extract is a bioflavonoid-rich, potent extract, which is used for fighting free radicals and maintaining capillary health. It is very similar to grape seed extract, with a high content of proanthocyanidins. Proanthocyanidins are found in many foods, but freezing, cooking and canning deactivate them.

Free radicals do damage in the capillaries in two ways: (1) by inactivating a compound called alpha 1-antitripsin, whose role is to restrain the enzymes that break down collagen, elastin and hyaluronic acid; and (2) by turning the fats in the cell membranes rancid (lipid peroxidation). Proanthocyanidins protect both the alpha 1-antitripsin and the lipids by neutralizing the specific types of free radicals most likely to damage them, and may also directly inhibit the damaging enzymes.

Collagen, elastin and hyaluronic acid make up much of the inner wall and supporting matrix of the capillaries. When they are in good condition the capillaries stretch to let red blood cells through more narrow spaces and do not let the fluid (plasma) in the blood leak out. Proanthocyanidins have shown a marked tendency to accumulate in tissues with high contents of glycosaminoglycans (complex amino sugars), such as capillary walls and skin. This may also apply to cartilage and synovial fluid. Proanthocyanidins have also shown antimutagenic effects in vitro at high concentrations (250 mcg/ml).

Proanthocyanidins (also known as leucoanthocyanidins) are a form of polyphenol, which is in turn a form of bioflavonoid. Proanthocyanidins are at least 15 to 25 times more powerful than vitamin E in neutralizing the iron and oxygen species of free radicals that attack lipids.

THERAPEUTIC USES

- poor distribution of microcirculatory blood flow in the brain and heart
- altered capillary fragility and permeability (e,g, in diabetes mellitus)
- chronic arterial/venous insufficiency in the extremities
- altered platelet aggregation and other characteristics of blood flow in capillaries
- breakdown in the elastic fibers of the capillaries (collagen and elastin) due to free radical and enzyme action
- microangiopathy of the retina, edema of the lymph nodes, and varicose veins

TOXICITY, CAUTIONS & CONTRAINDICATIONS

Proanthocyanidins are almost completely non-toxic both in acute dosage and long-term dosage. They have no potential for causing mutations or birth defects and have no adverse effect on fertility, pregnancy or nursing.

QUERCETIN

DESCRIPTION

Quercetin is a flavonoid found in the barks and rinds of many plants. A study in The Netherlands found the daily diet of 4,112 adults contained 23 mg of mixed flavonoids, including 16 mg of quercetin. Their most important sources were tea, onions, kale, endive and apples. Quercitin is the most active of the flavonoids. It is a yellow, crystalline derivative of several flavonoids.

Quercetin has anti-inflammatory, antiviral and anti-tumor properties. It inhibits the release of histamine and other inflammatory mediators (such as hyaluronidase and neutrophil lysosomal enzyme) from mast cells, basophils, neutrophils and macrophages. Its antioxidant action reduces damage from compounds that are released. Quercetin also inhibits smooth muscle contraction. It also inhibits many of the inflammatory products of fatty acid metabolism, especially phospholipase A2 and lipoxygenase enzyme production. This results in reduced formation of leucotrienes, which are 1,000 times more inflammatory than histamine, and are linked to asthma, psoriasis, atopic dermatitis, gout, ulcerative colitis, and possibly cancer. Quercetin was consistently effective in decreasing lipid peroxidation in stored whole red blood cells. An experiment with hydrogen peroxide-induced cytotoxicity and mutagenicity indicated that the catechol structure of polyphenols (0-dihydroxy) is critical to their effectiveness. In contrast, ferulic acid esters with an 0-methoxyphenol structure and alpha-tocopherol were ineffective. In a study of type-II estrogen binding sites in human meningiomas, quercetin competed with the tumors for binding sites on tritiated estradiols and inhibited in vitro the tumor cells' ability to incorporate bromodeoxyuridine. Quercetin treatment of tumor cell lines K562, Molt-4, Raji and MCAS caused condensation and fragmentation of nuclei, condensation of nuclear chromatin and fragmentation of DNA.

Usually 400 mg or more, is taken 20 minutes before each meal, unless the stomach is easily irritated, to a total of 1,200 to 2,000 mg per day or more, or as recommended by a health care professional.

THERAPEUTIC USES
- beneficial in cases of allergies, viruses (especially herpes type 1, para-influenza type 3, polio type 1 and respiratory syncytial)
- capillary fragility
- cancer prevention and treatment

TOXICITY, CAUTIONS & CONTRAINDICATIONS
No known toxicity. Quercetin is not mutagenic, but rather is strongly antimutagenic.

REISHI MUSHROOM

DESCRIPTION

Reishi mushroom, Ganoderma lucidum, is known as ling-zhi ("mushroom of immortality") in China. In Japan, it is called reishi mushroom or mannentake ("10,000 year old mushroom"). It is a basidomycetes and a polypore with pores under the cap instead of gills, and grows on the trunks or stumps of trees. Prune trees yield mushrooms with the highest level of ganoderic acid. Although it typically has a kidney shaped cap on a slightly twisted columnar stalk, it can also look like deer antlers and many other shapes. Reishi is distinguished by its brownish-red color with near-black and orange stripes, which are also highly variable. Ganoderma is the single most highly rated herb, in terms of multiple benefits and lack of side effects, in all of Traditional Chinese Medicine.

Of all the drugs and herbs listed in the "Shennong Medical Herbology," the ancient Chinese materia medica, was one which ranked higher than ginseng for its value in promoting health and well being. This famous medicinal herb, ling-zhi, was actually not an herb but a variety of fungus, belonging to the ganoderma genus. Among the large number of species in this botanical genus, "Red Ling-zhi" or Ganoderma lucidum, is the most popular and medicinally effective.

For over 2000 years, ling-zhi has been highly recommended as a valuable remedy by Chinese medicine practitioners. Highly regarded by the Chinese people as the "Medicine of Kings," it grows in the forest in very small quantities. Because of its rarity and preciousness, ling-zhi is also known as "the herb of good fortune."

Ling-zhi can be taken daily for long periods without any adverse side effects. Long-term use can help normalize body functions, empower the immune system to fight disease, and stabilize the internal environment. For example, both ling-zhi and ginseng are able to lower the blood pressure of a hypertensive patient and raise that of a hypotensive patient. Each of these has the ability to normalize body function. However, much depends on the quality and concentration, as poor quality or low concentration may not achieve the desired effect with either.

Its antiviral effects have been tested empirically in cases such as hepatitis B, HIV, chicken pox, herpes zoster, herpes genitalis, herpes labialis and mumps. In cases of chickenpox, the rash and severity of the disease may be greatly reduced when a high dose of reishi is started when the rash first appears. In herpes genitalis, the period of remission may be longer and the severity greatly reduced. Here too, the response is dose related.

The proteins in reishi mushrooms contain all the essential amino acids and most of the commonly occurring non-essential amino acids and amides. The fatty acids are largely unsaturated, and reishi are rich in vitamins (especially B3, B5, C and D) and minerals (especially calcium, phosphorous and iron). Ganoderma has the most active polysaccharides (long chains of sugars) among medicinal plant sources. Ganoderma is the only known source of a group of triterpenoides known as ganderic acids, which have a molecular structure similar to steroid hormones. A study of nine edible medicinal mushrooms connected their anti-tumor activity to polysaccharides and fatty substances that were probably ergosterols. Ganoderma also neutralized free radicals such as carbon tetrachloride and ethionine in animal livers, reversing fatty infiltration.

THERAPEUTIC USES
- hepatoprotective effect
- chronic bronchitis and cough
- anti-inflammatory effects without gastric side effects

- significantly lowered serum cholesterol but had no effect on triglycerides in studies
- anti-tumor effect
- essential hypertension
- potentially useful in auto-immune disorders, heart disease, and HIV infection
- increase non-specific immune function
- lengthen periods of remission and reduce severity of episodes of genital herpes

TOXICITY, CAUTIONS & CONTRAINDICATIONS

None. High doses of powdered reishi mushroom may lead to loosening of the stools, dry mouth, skin rash, or slight digestive upset. Extracts have been designed to reduce these adverse effects.

RESVERATOL

DESCRIPTION

Findings from published scientific literature indicates that reseveratol may be the most effective plant extract for maintaining optimal health. Red wine contains reseveratol, but the quantity varies depending on where the grapes are grown, the time of harvest, and other factors. After more than two years of relentless research, a standardized resveratol extract is now available as a dietary supplement. This whole grape extract contains a spectrum of polyphenol that are naturally contained in red wine such as proanthocyandins, anthocyanin, flavonoids, etc.

High concentrations of reservatol, (found to have anti-cloting effects and an ability to reduce fat deposits in animal livers) have been indentified in grape skins.

In addition, other important compounds have been identified in grape skins and grape seeds, powerful antioxidant factors called proanthocyanidins and polyphenols are found in large supply and are believed to prevent oxidation of LDL cholesterol (a major factor in heart disease). It is because of the strong antioxidant effect-some reports say 20-50 times stronger than Vitamin C and E that this result is accomplished. Wine drinkers, for example, tend to stay thinner, to exercise more, and to spend more time relaxing and socializing, all of which may have positive health benefits in and of themselves. Drinking too much mine or any alcoholic beverage has a definite down side. Numerous studies suggest t that consuming more than two drinks a day over the long term can raise blood pressure in some people and increase the risk for stroke and other diseases. However the standardized extract from red grape skin called reservetol is a perfect substitute of drinking wine.

TOXICITY, CAUTIONS, CONTRAINDICATIONS

No known toxicity

SAFED MUSLI

ORIGIN:
India

DESCRIPTION:
It is being used in Ayurvedic and Unani medicines, and has been for centuries, in India and the Indian subcontinent.It is used for debility and poor vitality. The plant is very small and short.

It is a medicinal plant, which is found in the Eastern - Southern part of India, more than the Northern part of India. It is a pretty herb of 2 feet high.

TYPES OF SAFED MUSLI:
There are 8 types of Safed Musli.
1. Chlorophytum borivillianum
2. Chlorophytum arundinaceum
3. Chlorophytum tuberocum
4. Chlorophytum malabericum
5. Chlorophytum attenuatum
6. Chlorophytum breviscapum
7. Asparagus filicinus
8. A gonoclados

THERAPEUTICS USES:
Its tubers are used in Ayurvedic medicine . It contains about 30% alkaloids, Natural steroid saponin (10-20%), polysaccaroids (40 to 45%), carbohydrates and proteins (5% to 7%). White Musli or Safed Musli is used for preparation of a health tonic in general and sexual debilities. As it is very rich in glycosides, It works very well in curing impotency.

TOXICITY:
Not known, no reported adverse effects.

SEA CUCUMBER

DESCRIPTION

Sea cucumbers are marine animals with elongated, tubular bodies, found in all seas of the world at all depths, usually lying on the ocean bottom on its flattened side. They are classified in the class Holothuridea of the phylum Echinodermata.

Trepang is a Malay word, referring to cooked, dried and smoked sea cucumbers, and Malaysians consider it to be a delicacy. In the Indian and Pacific Oceans, primarily in southern Japan, the Philippines and Indonesia, approximately 25 to 30 species are made into trepang and are eaten. It is generally used as a soup base. Sea cucumbers have been harvested for at least 1,000 years and are marketed in Asia, the USA and other countries. Sea cucumbers are also revered as aphrodisiacs in the Far East. Some suggest that many health problems and disorders can be prevented by using sea cucumber. It is the marine organisms' defensive toxin that may be useful in treating some human diseases. Sea cucumber has anti-inflammatory properties reportedly 25 times more powerful than aspirin. According to research done in 1992 at the University of Queensland, Australia, it is a potent antiarthritic. Sea cucumber is broadly used in homeopathic remedies.

THERAPEUTIC USES

- many types of arthritis
- tendinitis
- sports injuries
- joint pains

SHARK CARTILAGE

DESCRIPTION

Shark fin soup is a traditional Chinese specialty dish, claimed traditionally to have enormous health benefits. The truth in the claim is substantiated by a simple fact: sharks rarely, if ever, get cancer. Having existed largely unchanged for over 300 million years, they have a cartilaginous instead of a calcified bony skeleton. Based on research, it is thought to be this large amount of cartilage, 68 percent of their gross weight, that gives sharks their apparent immunity to cancer.

Current research illustrates that shark cartilage will inhibit the formation of new blood capillary networks needed by growing tumors for their nutrient requirements. Without a capillary network to feed a tumor and remove its wasted products, a tumor or metastasis will not grow. Without new and replacement capillaries, tumors will slowly shrink in size. A widely accepted theory, developed and published by scientists at Harvard University, shows that a tumor will never become larger than two cubic millimeters (the size of a small pencil point) if a new blood network is prevented from forming to nourish it. This is the basis on which shark cartilage works against numerous diseases.

Recently, scientists at the Massachusetts Institute of Technology (MIT) published findings that an extract of shark cartilage contains a protein substance that strongly inhibits the development of new blood networks. This inhibitor, identified by the same research team, is a large (or macro-) protein molecule found most abundantly in shark cartilage. All cartilage contains this protein inhibitor, called an anti-angioneogenesis factor, but published data clearly establishes that shark cartilage has 1,000 times more of this inhibitor than any other common type of cartilage.

Based on these published works and numerous studies carried out at the prestigious Institute Jules Bordet in Brussels, the University of Arizona Cancer Research Center, and by scientists associated with the University of Miami School of Medical, it has been shown that orally administered dry shark cartilage is most effective.

Also, a nontoxic product made from 100 percent pure shark cartilage, properly processed with a very high concentration of the inhibitor, is now available. Initial test results on animals and humans, plus the simplicity of the theory behind its method of action, have created much excitement in the medical field. Important clinical trials on cancer are ongoing to augment the animal studies on cancer.

Extensive research on the pain associated with arthritis and its effect on mobility has been conducted on dogs and on humans in both Belgium and Florida. The human studies showed reductions in pain and increases in mobility, all within two to three weeks of beginning the oral daily administration of dry, pulverized shark cartilage. The dog studies, which eliminated the placebo effect, used 16 dogs with severe, incapacitating arthritis. These dogs demonstrated increased mobility after just 14 days of daily shark cartilage treatment with food (1g of cartilage for each 15 pounds of body weight). Criteria such as ease of action and jumping over obstacles were measured and recorded. All dogs improved significantly, though this improvement was lost when the cartilage administration was stopped for two weeks. By reintroducing the cartilage feeding, all the gains were reestablished, even with lower dosage levels.

Most people who have well-formed blood networks will not need new vascularization unless a blood vessel-dependent malady such as a tumor begins to develop. Deny the network, and you will probably stop the tumor.

THERAPEUTIC USES

- helping control tumor or metastasic growth by inhibiting new vascularization
- possible use in treating the inflammation and pain associated with degenerative and rheumatoid arthritis
- possible use in diabetic retinopathy
- possible use in treating psoriasis

TOXICITY, CAUTIONS & CONTRAINDICATIONS

Pregnant women and people who have recently experienced a heart attack (and must develop new blood vessels in the heart) should obviously not take shark cartilage.

SHARK LIVER OIL

DESCRIPTION

Shark liver oil has been used by fisherman for centuries as a folk remedy for relieving general debility, for healing wounds, sores, irritations of the respiratory tract and the alimentary canal, and for reducing lymph node swelling. Shark liver oil from Greenland is rich in alkyglycerols, which are naturally found in breast milk and in bone marrow. That from Alaska, is rich in vitamins A and D, and in essential omega-3 fatty acids. Greenland shark liver oil contains the highest level of alkylgylycerols found in nature. The active ingredients are predominantly esters of selachyl-, chimyl-, and batyl-alcohol, and methoxy-substituted compounds of glycerol. There are 16 known alkylgylycerols, with shark liver oil containing the most concentrated source.

Alkylgylycerols are involved in the production of white blood cells. Shark liver oil was found to stimulate the body's immune system, increasing antibodies, leukocytes and thrombocytes. In particular, it was found to increase the survival rate of cervical cancer patients, and to reduce radiation-induced injuries of leukopenia and thrombocytopenia. Recent research has also shown that alkylgylycerols have antibiotic and anti-fungal effects, can speed up the healing of wounds, and can increase the excretion of mercury.

TOXICITY, CAUTIONS & CONTRAINDICATIONS

No known toxicity.

SHILAJIT

DESCRIPTION

Shilajit is a classical Ayurvedic Medicine used in diverse clinical conditions. It has been proposed to arrest aging, to induce rejuvenation, and to improve memory, the major attributes of Ayurveda rasayana (antiaging) herbs. Some recent scientific studies have reported on the importance of Shilajit in different pathological conditions and as a possible psychotropic agent. Shilajit is initially a blackish brown, sticky exudation of variable consistency with the odor of cow urine. It is derived from the rocky faces and crevices of different formations in the Himalayan mountains of Nepal, at altitudes between 1,000-5,000 meters. Subsequently, it is prepared through an ancient series of processes into a powder. It is an eminent multimineral preparation frequently used in Ayurvedic medicine for the management of various disorders. The Charaka Samhita, the oldest book on Ayurveda, in confirming the efficacy of this multimineral states that there is almost no curable health problems which cannot be managed by Shilajit administration.

In Ayurveda, Shilajit is known as Silajitu or Silajitu Dhatuja. In English, it is known as Black Bitumen. The Latin name for Shilajit is Asphaltum Panjainum. In Nepal, it is called Silajita.

Shilajit in the view of ancient authors mentioned earlier, is a derivative of various metals e.g. Gold, Silver, Copper, Iron, Lead and Zinc. According to available descriptions, this mineral can be classified:

    A. According to its source and constituents.
    B. According to its odor.
    C. According to the process involved during purification.

Given its descriptions in ancient Ayurvedic literature, Shilajit was likely considered a source of multiple minerals.

The origin of the minerals is said to be from the mountain rocks in summer months. Most of the Ayurvedic texts have considered it as an exudate from the metal-containing rocks (e.g. Gold, Silver, Copper and black iron), which emerged after being melted by the heat exposure of the sun's rays during summer.

THERAPEUTIC USES

- Shilajit has been used for ages in Ayurvedic medicine and other traditional medicines in the treatment of bronchial asthma, diabetes, impotency, genitourinary disorders, wound healing and stomach ulcers.
- People in the Himalayas use Shilajit to combat cold stress and as a tonic.

TOXICITY, CAUTIONS AND CONTRAINDICATIONS

Shilajit is a well tolerated, safe and non-toxic multiple mineral. If desired, it can be given for fairly long periods without any known danger of toxic effects on any organ or tissue of the body.

SHIITAKE MUSHROOM

DESCRIPTION

Shiitake is the Japanese name for this mushroom, which is simply called "black mushroom" in Chinese restaurant menus. It grows on the trunks or stumps of trees. Like certain seaweeds, shiitake is an important part of the diets of many people in Asia, particularly China and Japan. However, shiitake is traditionally used as a tea by those who want to gain its formidable immune-enhancing benefits. For this purpose, some say the mushrooms must be boiled in a covered container for a minimum of two hours and then consumed as a tea, while others suggest steeping an ounce of chopped, dried shiitake in a pint of boiled water. However it is prepared, shiitake mushroom tea or extract offers remarkable anti-tumor benefits which are particularly helpful in cases of HIV infection and AIDS. In this case, it is more reliable to buy the extract form from your health food store and take concentrated shiitake as a dietary supplement.

The proteins in shiitake contain all of the essential amino acids, and most of the commonly occurring non-essential amino acids and amides. The fatty acids are largely unsaturated, and shiitake is rich in vitamins and minerals. Key therapeutic substances include the glucans, a major constituent of the cell walls. Shiitake yields lentinan, a beta-1,3-linked glucan polysacharride with a molecular weight of one million. This activates the alternative complement pathway, stimulating the macrophages, thus inhibiting tumor growth. Thus it stimulates the immune system, rather than directly acting on the tumor. Because of its large molecular size, lentinan is not absorbed efficiently when taken orally, though some is absorbed. Shiitake is believed to stimulate interferon production. It significantly inhibits the toxic immunosuppresive effects of cancer drugs such as cyclocytidine when taken with them. Eritadenine, a purine alkaloid from shiitake, is similar to nucleotides in structure and lowers cholesterol in animal studies.

THERAPEUTIC USES
- helpful in some cancers
- cholesterol reduction
- counteracts some effects of diseases of the liver, such as hepatitis and cirrhosis
- improves immune response, including in those with AIDS

TOXICITY, CAUTIONS & CONTRAINDICATIONS
None known. Shiitake is highly edible and delicious.

SPIRULINA

DESCRIPTION

Spirulina is called a superfood because its nutrients are more concentrated than other foods, plants, grains or herbs. Spirulina is a microscopic blue-green algae. It is a vegetable plankton whose cells form the shape of a coiled spring (thus the name spirulina, which means "little spiral").

Spirulina provides protein, carbohydrates, vitamins, amino acids, protective pigments, and many other vital nutrients important in human health. In addition to its amazing ability to support human nutrition, spirulina has the potential to help relieve world hunger and renew the planet's ecosystem. It provides a means of more efficient land utilization for protein production as compared to meat production. Spirulina provides for more efficient water utilization as compared to other agricultural uses and is even more efficient at fixing carbon and releasing oxygen into the atmosphere than trees.

Spirulina is a nutrient dense food. In contrast to the protein in meat, the protein found in spirulina is easily digested. Its benefit as a whole food includes all the essential amino acids, a high level of beta carotene (provitamin A), B vitamins, trace minerals, GLA, chlorophyll and other important micronutrients.

Amid reports of new viruses, drug-resistant bacteria and ineffective antibiotics, scientists are discovering the ability of certain foods to strengthen the immune system and prevent disease. The National Cancer Institute has identified compounds found in blue-green algae like spirulina as remarkably active against the AIDS virus. A Russian patent was awarded to spirulina as a medical food for improving the immunity of the "Children of Chernobyl" suffering from radiation illness. Reports from

HIV-positive patients and children with malnutrition show spirulina helps to boost the immune system.

Animal researchers are also realizing the power of spirulina. Through separate studies, scientists in North Carolina, Japan and China have discovered that small amounts of spirulina added to animal feed greatly help animals resist infections. Already widely used for aquaculture fish, shrimps, exotic pet birds and race horses, spirulina will soon be used in feeds for healthier chickens, turkeys and other animals.

As one of the oldest living plants on the planet, spirulina has been a source of food for some cultures for centuries. Spirulina is 60 percent all-vegetable protein, higher than any other food. It contains vitamin B12, iron and the rare essential fatty acid, GLA. Its dark green color comes from phytonutrients such as carotenes, chlorophylls and phytocyanin. Spirulina has been consumed by millions of people in the US and 40 other countries for over 15 years.

Spirulina is sold in tablets, capsules and powder. The dark green powder can be blended into fruit and milk drinks or added to recipes to boost nutritional value. Research suggests six tablets or one teaspoon of powder a day can increase health and energy.

SUPEROXIDE DISMUTASE (SOD)

DESCRIPTION

Human beings cannot live without breathing the air, which contains a sufficient amount of oxygen to sustain life. A fact much less well known is that not all oxygen atoms support life. Some are actually quite destructive. These unhealthy oxygen atoms are unbalanced and constitute the most common free radical known. Characterized by having an unpaired electron in its molecular structure, this oxygen free radical, called superoxide, is quite capable of causing cell damage.

Enzymes are necessary to trigger bodily functions, but are not a part of the resulting molecular structures. Superoxide dismutase (SOD) is a protein, an enzyme, found in all body cells. Originally known as erythrocuprein, it was discovered in the liver and other organs of cows and is now available as a supplement. SOD's apparent mode of operating is to fight the devastating effects of the "superoxide" radical, a substance which the body constantly creates. The importance of SOD is so paramount for the protection of our cells, that it represents a substantial proportion of the proteins manufactured by the body. In brief, SOD keeps oxygen under control.

Dismutation (deactivation) is the process by which the free radical is transformed into stable oxygen and semi-stable hydrogen peroxide (called semi-stable because it eventually breaks down into more free radicals). This alteration of the free radicals prevents what might otherwise be irreparable cell damage, which would otherwise result in rapid aging, degeneration and death.

Nature accompanies SOD with catalase, a second dismuting enzyme, to remove hydrogen peroxide and leave water and oxygen in its place. Integrated in all red blood cells, catalase removes hydrogen peroxide from our tissues, preventing both cell damage and, more importantly, the formation of other, more toxic, free radicals. In nature, and in the body, SOD and catalase always coexist. The natural interaction between these two antioxidant enzymes constitutes the most effective system of free radical control in our bodies. SOD administered without catalase still does some good, because the body's own catalase dismutes some of the hydrogen peroxide. However, SOD with catalase, in tablets or drops, is better than plain SOD.

Superoxide free radicals initiate the breakdown of the lubricating synovial fluid in the joints, causing friction and eventual inflammation. For this reason the attention of clinical SOD research has been focused primarily on inflammatory processes triggered by superoxide free radicals such as arthritis, bursitis and gout. Deficiency in SOD/catalase is the most notorious nutritional factor in most inflammatory processes. Recent applications of SOD/catalase enhancing foods have also proven to be extremely useful as a pre- and postoperative supplement, which stimulates recovery and reduces convalescent periods remarkably.

One of the most exiting things about SOD (among all its other qualities) is the discovery that it slows down the aging process. Free radicals speed up the aging of the body by attaching to the body's supportive tissue, collagen. The collagen tissues become less flexible, even rigid, and the signs of old age begin to appear. The limbs become stiff, the skin begins to wrinkle, and unhealthy fatty deposits in the arterial walls increase. The walls of the arteries become rigid and hypertension often results. SOD prevents or at least considerably slows the process of deterioration.

Considering the powerful link between free radicals and many health problems, supplements that enhance SOD and catalase activity in the body offer tremendous potential in the field of preventive nutrition.

TONGKAT ALI

DESCRIPTION:

Supporting, healthy testosterone levels, Tongkat Ali (Eurycoma longifolia) has an ancient reputation as an aphrodisiac in Malaysia and Indonesia, where its known as Pasak Bumi. Its name means "Ali's staff or walking stick" in reference to its effects on male sexuality.

A study by the Forest Research Institute of Malaysia (FRIM) showed that the Eurycoma Longifolia Jack or Tongkat Ali (Pasak Bumin) contains, anti-oxidant properties, a high level of SOD (Superoxide Dismutase), an anti-oxidant enzyme. The aqueous and methanol extracts of Tongkat Ali has an effect of scavenging superoxide and lipid peroxidation. This showed that Tongkat Ali could inhibit the chain reaction of free radicals that could be harmful to the tissues of the body.

Research has shown that Eurycoma Longifolia Jack contains several phytochemicals (plant chemicals) that support healthy testosterone levels (the sex hormone) required for the male sexual functions. It also supports healthy sexual organs and mental alertness.

Traditionally Eurycoma Longifolia Jack (Tongkat Ali) is used to
• Support general health and vitality
• Support sexual drive in men
• Support healthy energy levels
• Support healthy blood circulation

TOXICITY:

not known

TYROSINE

DESCRIPTION

Acutely stressful situations can disrupt behavior and deplete brain neurotransmitters. Using a double-blind placebo controlled crossover design, U.S. soldiers were tested to see whether tyrosine supplementation would protect them from some of the adverse consequences of a 4.5 hour exposure to cold and high altitude. Tyrosine significantly decreased symptoms, adverse moods, and performance impairments in response to these environmental conditions. The researchers assessed symptoms, mood, cognitive performance, and reaction time since cold and high altitude environments produce a variety of adverse effects. The performance tasks employed required maintaining sustained attention, applying prior knowledge to problems, processing spatial and verbal information, performing mathematical calculations, and making decisions. Performance on each task was defined as number of problems correct per minute. Choice reaction time was also measured. Tyrosine significantly reduced many adverse behavioral effects produced by exposure to cold and high altitude. Tyrosine, compared to placebo, significantly reduced symptoms of headache, coldness, distress, fatigue, muscular discomfort, and sleepiness. During exposure to the environmental stressors, tyrosine treatment also reduced dizziness, confusion, unhappiness, hostility, and tension.

The study was designed to investigate whether tryosine supplementation reduces cognitive impairment and physiological stress in humans exposed to a combination of mental and physical stressors. While performing stress-sensitive tasks, subjects were exposed to a stressor noise of 90 dB. Tyrosine was found to improve performance of cognitive tasks, which were performed one hour after administration. In addition, tyrosine decreased diastolic blood pressure 15 minutes after ingestion, while one hour after ingestion diastolic blood pressure was the same with tyrosine and placebo. As an environmental stressor, a continuous broadband noise with an intensity of 90 dB was induced. The noise consisted of a mixture of sounds including factory, traffic and trains. A word-color choice test called Stroop Task was conducted. The number of errors and response time were recorded. A short-term memory test involving numbers called Digit Span was also conducted. Significant tyrosine treatment effects were found for both of these two tasks. The data from the Stroop Task test revealed that subjects performed this task faster with tyrosine. With respect to the Digit Span test, the number of correct responses was higher with tyrosine.

THERAPEUTIC USES

The present results indicate that the administration of tyrosine improved cognitive function under stress.

TOXICITY, CAUTIONS & CONTRAINDICATIONS

No known toxicity

WHEAT GERM OIL

DESCRIPTION

Wheat germ oil is a nutritionally rich vegetable oil made from the germ portion of fresh, high quality wheat kernels by a cold process, which preserves valuable nutrients, essential factors, flavor and aroma.

Wheat germ oil is an excellent source of essential fatty acids, particularly ALA and linoleic acid, of natural vitamin E (alpha and beta tocopherols), and octacosanol. With its low saturated fat content and its high nutritional quality, it is also an attractive substitute for heavily processed vegetable oils used in foods such as salad oils, batter mixes, and cake mixes.

Wheat germ oil is a valuable source of essential fatty acids, including linoleic acid and alpha-linolenic acid, as well as natural vitamin E complex. Fatty acids such as linoleic and linolenic acids, which are essential in the diet, provide the building blocks for a variety of structural lipids, hormones, prostaglandins, and other polyunsaturated acids used as energy sources. Octacosanol, one of the principle factors responsible for the reported beneficial effects of wheat germ oil, has been demonstrated to improve strength, stamina and reaction time. The vitamin E content is due to the naturally occurring tocopherols that are abundant in unrefined, pure wheat germ oil and is not an additive.

TOXICITY, CAUTIONS & CONTRAINDICATIONS

No known toxicity.

INDEX
OF
HERBS

ADHATODA VASICA

ORIGIN
India, Sri Lanka

PART OF PLANT USED
Leaves

DESCRIPTION
The medicinal properties of Adhatoda vasica Nees (Order: Acanthaceae), have been known in India and several other countries for thousands of years. The plant has been recommended by Ayurvedic physicians for the management of various types of respiratory disorders.

The leaves of the plant contain an essential oil and the quinazoline alkaloids vasicine, vasicinone and deoxyvasicine. The roots contain vasicinolone, vasicol, peganine and 2'-hydroxy-4-glucosyl-oxychalcone. The flowers contain Beta-sitosterol-D-glucoside, kaempferol and its glucosides, as well as the bioflavonoid, quercetin.

The leaves are used in the treatment of respiratory disorders in Ayurveda. Research over the last three decades revealed that the alkaloids vasicine and vasicinone, present in the leaves, possess respiratory stimulant activity. Vasicine, at low concentrations, induced bronchodilation and relaxation of the tracheal muscles. At high concentrations, vasicine offered significant protection against histamine-induced bronchospasm in guinea pigs. Vasicinone, the auto-oxidation product of vasicine, has been reported to cause bronchodilation both in vitro and in vivo. In another study, vasicine showed appreciable bronchodilatory effect and marked respiratory stimulant activities whereas vasicinone showed relaxation of the tracheal muscles in vitro and bronchoconstriction in vivo. Of the two alkaloids, vasicinone is more potent than vasicine, with antiasthmatic activity comparable to that of disodium cromoglycate.

TRADITIONAL AND OTHER THERAPEUTIC USES

- asthma
- cough
- respiratory ailments

TOXICITY, CAUTIONS AND CONTRAINDICATIONS

Adhatoda vasica has very low toxicity and reported side effects are rare.

ALFALFA
(Medicago sativa)

ORIGIN
Believed to have originated in central and western Asia

PARTS OF PLANT USED
Leaves and flowers

DESCRIPTION
Also know as "buffalo herb" and "sweet lucerne," alfalfa grows in dry fields, in sandy wastes, and along some roadsides. It reaches a height of one to two feet and has bluish purple flowers from June through August (although there is a variety with yellow flowers that crosses freely with the purple and produces innumerable shades of lilac, green, cream and even white flowers). The leaves, petals, and flowers are commonly used to treat stomach and blood disorders. One of the richest sources of trace minerals, alfalfa is high in calcium, iron, magnesium, phosphorus, potassium, and chlorine, as well as vitamin K.

Alfalfa is a perennial plant with soft green compound leaves and yellow to purplish-blue flowers. It is a forage legume plant belonging to the pea family, Leguminosae. Alfalfa is grown throughout the world, in a variety of climactic conditions. It thrives in loamy, fertilized and watered home gardens with deep, well-drained, nonacidic soil. It does best with ample supplies of phosphorus and potassium. Varieties of alfalfa are grown from the equator up to as 60°N latitude.

Alfalfa has been used as an herbal remedy since before recorded history. The crushed dried leaves and/or kidney shaped seeds are brewed as a tea. Some find the spinach taste of alfalfa tea to be unpleasant. Anise, citrus, mint or honey may be added to improve the tea's flavor. Tender alfalfa sprouts are often added to salads and sandwiches.

TRADITIONAL AND OTHER THERAPEUTIC USES

- possessing natural anti-inflammatory properties, used to treat gout and arthritis
- soothe active peptic ulcer disease
- effective in lowering blood sugar in diabetics and may stimulate insulin production (according to some recent research)
- useful in cases of hemorrhaging and fungal infections
- available in liquid form as a mineral supplement

TOXICITY, CAUTIONS AND CONTRAINDICATIONS

Alfalfa seeds and sprouts have a large amount of L-canavanine. Because of its reported connection with initiating lupus in primates, some authorities feel the seeds and sprouts should be avoided, and that all alfalfa should be avoided in those with lupus and other connective tissue diseases.

ARTICHOKE
(Cynara scolymus)

PARTS OF PLANT USED
Flower heads, leaves, and roots

DESCRIPTION
The flower head of the globe artichoke is used as a common food. The artichoke head, leaves and root contain several active components important for liver, kidney and gall bladder complaints.

Artichokes contain cynarin and scolymoside, which have been shown to stimulate bile secretion. Cynarin also has been reported to lower cholesterol and triglyceride levels. Artichoke also has some diuretic activities and has been used for kidney diseases and proteinuria.

TRADITIONAL AND OTHER THERAPEUTIC USES
- improves sluggish liver, increasing bile secretion
- relieves poor digestion
- fights atherosclerosis
- lowers elevated tryglycerides, elevated cholesterol
- kidney diseases and especially proteinuria

TOXICITY, CAUTIONS AND CONTRAINDICATIONS
There is no known toxicity.

ASHWAGANDHA
(Withania somnifera)

ORIGIN
India

PARTS OF PLANT USED
Roots and leaves

DESCRIPTION
Long ago, before the births of Buddhism, Yoga and Christianity, ashwagandha was used as a healing herb in India. Today, after thousands of years of continuous use, ashwagandha is regarded as one of the most valuable Ayurvedic medicinal plants.

Sometimes called "Indian Ginseng," ashwagandha has been used in a number of forms to treat a huge variety of physical maladies. The roots and leaves of the plant are prepared traditionally in a number of ways, including as a powder, decoction, oil, and poultice. These have been suggested for the cure of various diseases such as leprosy, nervous disorders, intestinal infections, sexually transmitted diseases, rheumatism, and emaciation. Also, it is popularly used by physicians in India as an aphrodisiac.

After long use in India, ashwagandha has been introduced to the West and has enjoyed a very enthusiastic reception in the scientific community. Its use has been mentioned as an amebacide, anodyne, bactericide, diuretic, emmenagogue, fungicide, sedative, and tonic. Also noted was ashwagandha's use in folk medicine against arthritis, asthma, cancer, candidiasis, colds, cough, cystitis, debility, diarrhea, fever, gynecopathy, hiccups, hypertension, inflammation, lumbago, nausea, piles, proctitis, psoriasis, rheumatism, ringworm, scabies, senility, small pox, sores, syphilis, tuberculosis, tumors, typhoid, and wounds.

While it may be a bit too strong to say that ashwagandha prevents or cures everything from hiccups to cancer, it no doubt has impressive adaptogenic properties. With a program of good nutrition, it can boost both immunity and endurance.

TRADITIONAL AND OTHER THERAPEUTIC USES
- increases resistance to stress
- improves physical endurance

TOXICITY, CAUTIONS AND CONTRAINDICATIONS
No known toxicity or side effects; used in India for over 2,500 years.

ASTRAGALUS
(Astragalus membranaceus)

ORIGIN
China, Taiwan, Korea

PART OF PLANT USED
Roots

DESCRIPTION
In traditional Chinese medicine, astragalus, known to the Chinese as huang qi and in North America as "milk vetch root," has demonstrated striking results in stimulating the immune system. In fact, it is one of the most powerful immune system boosters known.

A popular way to prepare astragalus is to put one teaspoon of the root into 1-1/2 pints of water in a covered container, and slowly boil for 20 to 30 minutes. Allow to cool slowly in the container, keeping it covered. Drink one cup at a time, twice daily. Also available as the supplement, Radix astragali, "Yellow Leader," or as part of a Chinese herbal mixture called qiang gan ruan jian tang, astragalus is recognized in traditional Chinese medicine for its importance as a tonic herb. First recorded in an herbal text over 2,000 years ago, and still one of the most popular herbs in China, astragalus is prized for its ability to increase ch'i (qi), or "life energy." This, in turn, helps to overcome fatigue, control diabetes, lower blood pressure, and treat coronary heart disease and anemia. Astragalus' properties include antiviral, antibacterial, immunostimulatory, anti-inflammatory, and as an energy tonic. It promotes drainage of abscesses and cysts.

In scientific studies, astragalus membranaceus was screened for its immunomodulating activity and was found to augment the proliferation of mononuclear white blood cells (macrophages and lymphocytes) in vitro. Some studies on the effects of astragalus in cancer treatment have been very promising. It is one of the principal herbs being studied by scientists at the American Cancer Society. Research has shown that astragalus is valuable in strengthening the immune systems of cancer patients. Those who are receiving chemotherapy or radiation therapy have been shown to recover faster and for longer periods when they take astragalus during treatment.

With most medicines and some herbs, there are side effects and/or tolerances, which can be built up, so care and moderation need to be exercised when you use them. Astragalus, on the other hand, has a broad range of healthful results and is safe to use. Therefore, we would recommend it as a tea or supplement for healthy people to maintain their health, as well as for those with specific maladies, which this herb has been used to treat.

Astragalus contains a unique isoflavone, termed 4' hydroxy-3'-methoxyisoflavone 7-sug, which has some pharmacological actions upon digestion. Other ingredients of astragalus include the triterpenoid saponins (astragalosides, astramembrannins), which are analogous to the animal steroid hormones. Also important in astragalus are the numerous polysaccharides, which have shown in pharmacological experiments to enhance the activity of the immune system, particularly NK and T-cell function and increased interferon production.

TRADITIONAL AND OTHER THERAPEUTIC USES

- classically to strengthen the wei qi, or defensive energy, and to "warm" the exterior
- increase resistance to disease and infections
- hepatitis, HIV infection and AIDS, and other viral conditions
- hypertension and peripheral vascular diseases

- possible uses for myasthenia gravis, immune depletion in cancer patients, ischemia

TOXICITY, CAUTIONS AND CONTRAINDICATIONS

No known toxicity.

AVENA SATIVA
(Wild Oat Seed)

DESCRIPTION

Avena sativa (Wild Oats) is a botanical extract that has traditionally been used to increase strength in the body, mind, and spirit. References to the sexual stimulating effects of oats have been found up to 200 years ago in the German Pharmacopocia. Modern studies at the Institute For Advanced Study of Human Sexuality have shown that Avena sativa helps improve interest in sex, acting as an aphrodesiac. Some research specializing in Sexology was conducted as a pilot study of Avena sativa. The volunteers in the study expressed interest in improving their sexual response. Factors that interfere with sexual performance include stress, limited time, age, lack of desire and sexual dysfunction. Their dysfunction/dissatisfaction ranged from male impotence and female lack of desire to inability to respond sexually. The volunteers, ages 22-64 years, consisted of 20 men and 20 women who were given a 300 mg capsule of Avena sativa extract; which they took three days a week for six weeks. Men experienced a 22% increase in genital sensation and women experienced a 15% increase in genital sensation. Men experienced a 36% increase in the frequency of orgasms and women experienced a 29% increase in the frequency of orgasms.

The pilot study showing Avena sativa's role as an aphrodisiac led the Institute to conduct further studies. Another study group of 120 volunteers was drawn from a larger pool that expressed interest in sexual enhancement. Avena sativa 300mg capsules were given to Group 1 for 28 days and then replaced by a placebo for an additional 28 days. Group 2 did this in reverse. The male volunteers reported an increased sex drive, enhanced firmness in erection and more pleasure during sex when taking Avena sativa vs. the placebo.

Avena sativa works with testosterone to enhance sexuality. Adequate levels of testosterone are essential in sexual functioning of both males and females. Scientists have found that with advancing age, testosterone becomes bound with various compounds within the body. Researchers at the Institute have discovered that Avena sativa works by freeing up testosterone. When testosterone is free, nature takes its course by stimulating sexual interest in both men and women. Thus, Avena sativa nutritionally supports your body's chemistry to enhance sexual desire, sensation and performance.

TRADITIONAL AND OTHER THERAPEUTIC USES
- improves sexual performance by maximizing your testosterone level
- reduces recovery time between sexual events and increase sexual intensity of activities
- increases sexual desire
- increases orgasms

TOXICITY, CAUTIONS AND CONTRAINDICATIONS
None noted.

BILBERRY
(Vaccinium murtillus L.)

ORIGIN
Europe (wild)

PART OF PLANT USED
Fresh fruit

DESCRIPTION
Bilberry is a perennial shrub native to northern Europe. It is similar to American bilberry but contains higher quantities of useful constituents for visual improvement. Over 15 different potent antioxidants have been found in bilberry. It is effective in the treatment of circulation disorders, varicose veins, and other venous and arterial disorders. It protects veins and arteries by stabilizing the endothelial cells, increasing the synthesis of collagen, and preventing the aggregation and adherence of platelets to endothelial surfaces. Likely because of these positive vascular effects, studies have shown that bilberry can be helpful in diabetic retinopathy. Bilberry has also been found to stimulate rhodopsin production.

TRADITIONAL AND OTHER THERAPEUTIC USES
- varicose veins and other venous disorders
- improves vision and treats night blindness

TOXICITY, CAUTIONS AND CONTRAINDICATIONS
No known toxicity.

BLACK COHOSH
(Cimicifuga racemosa)

ORIGIN
North America, Europe

DESCRIPTION
Black cohosh is a common name for a North American perennial herb of the buttercup family (Ranunculaceae), also called "bugbane" or "black snake root." Like other members of the family, it has one or a few large leaves, with each being divided so as to appear to be many individual leaves.

The principal medicinal value of black cohosh is as a natural and safe alternative to hormone replacement therapy (HRT) in women undergoing menopause. Current HRT treatment includes a combination of estrogen and progesterone. There are a number of studies suggesting that HRT might result in increased risk of certain types of cancer, particularly breast cancer, and especially in those women already at risk because of a genetic predisposition. Although not conclusively proven, there is enough concern regarding increased cancer risk that a safe and natural herbal alternative, which can produce the same reduction of menopausal symptoms, would be a wise choice.

The most widely used, and only thoroughly studied, natural approach to menopause is black cohosh standardized to contain 1 mg of triterpenes, calculated as 27-deoxyactein, per tablet. Clinical studies have shown black cohosh to relieve not only hot flashes, but also depression and vaginal atrophy. The VGA, the German equivalent to the FDA in the United States, includes no contraindications or limitations for the use of black cohosh in tumor patients. Therefore, black cohosh can offer a suitable natural alternative to HRT, especially where HRT is contraindicated, such as in women with a history of breast, endometrial, or liver cancers, unexplained uterine bleeding, liver disease, history of deep vein inflammation or blood clots, cerebrovascular or coronary artery disease, or diabetes with vascular involvement.

Black cohosh has been shown to produce symptomatic relief comparable to that of HRT without the risk of serious side effects.

TOXICITY, CAUTIONS AND CONTRAINDICATIONS

Detailed toxicology studies have been performed on black cohosh. No teratogenic, mutagenic, or carcinogenic effects have been noted.

BORAGE OIL
(Borago officinalis)

ORIGIN
Eastern Mediterranean

PART OF PLANT USED
Oil from the seed

DESCRIPTION
Often grown for bee feeding, salads, and beverage flavoring, starflower (Borago officinalis) is a 60-centimeter (2-foot), hairy, annual plant with large, rough, oblong leaves and loose, drooping clusters of star-like, bright blue flowers. It belongs to the family of Boraginaceae. The five bright yellow stamens form a cone at the star's center. Flowers are sometimes white or rose colored, and flowering stalks are usually reddish. Native to the eastern Mediterranean region, it was used by the ancient Greeks. It is cultivated today in various parts of Europe, Great Britain and North America.

The borage plant has a cool, cucumber-like taste and the leaves are cooked as a vegetable in Europe. Dried or fresh leaves are used in seasoning stews and soups. The translucent yellow edible oil produced from borage seed is used in supplements, dietetic foods, and cosmetics (skin solutions, ointments, creams, and shampoos).

Borage oil naturally contains a high quantity of the essential fatty acid, gamma linolenic acid (GLA). GLA is normally synthesized in the liver from dietary linoleic acid (LA). This reaction however is frequently deficient in many people because of interference by sugar, saturated fats, and trans-fatty acids (e.g. margarine). In addition the conversion requires vitamins B3, B6, and C as well as the minerals magnesium, zinc, and copper. Any deficiencies of these nutrients will affect the conversion.

As part of the Omega 6 series of essential fatty acids, GLA is the critical precursor to the Series 1 prostaglandins (PGE1) and other hormones in the body. The PGE1 series prostaglandins along with the PGE3 series protect the body against the deleterious effects of PGE2 series prostaglandins, such as high blood pressure, sticky platelets, inflammation, water retention, and lowered immune function. The series 2 prostaglandins are made from arachidonic acid, which is derived from consumption of excess animal products.

TRADITIONAL AND OTHER THERAPEUTIC USES
- helpful in reducing cholesterol
- benefits cystic fibrosis (daily dose of 1,500 mg borage oil containing 330 mg GLA)
- helpful in multiple sclerosis
- may benefit those with atherosclerosis and diabetes mellitus
- local application improves dermatitis, particularly infantile seborrhoeic dermatitis (ISD), eczema, and other skin conditions
- may decrease symptoms of premenstrual syndrome (PMS)
- effective in transepidermal water loss
- decreases blood pressure, therefore especially beneficial to hypertension patients
- historically, used to heal nose and throat ailments, and other vague problems such as madness and bad blood

TOXICITY, CAUTIONS AND CONTRAINDICATIONS
No known toxicity is associated with borage oil. Excess consumption can result in oily skin, an indication to decrease dosage.

BOSWELLA
(Boswella Serrata)

ORIGIN
India

PART OF PLANT USED
Gum resin

DESCRIPTION

Boswella serrata is a moderate to large branching tree, about 12 feet in height and three to four feet in girth. It is widely distributed throughout India, generally found in dry, hilly areas. The herbal product, Boswella, is the selectively fractionated principle obtained from the tree's gum resin. Its collection is restricted to certain parts of India and is carried out toward the end of October.

Used both internally as an herbal medicine and externally as a balm, Boswella offers relief without side effects for many arthritis sufferers. Contemporary researchers and physicians are validating the findings of medical texts more than 1,500 years old, which praise the anti-inflammatory and antiarthritic uses of the gummy extract. In a series of recent studies conducted at Indian government laboratories, the extract from Boswella serrata was found to be both safe and effective.

Researchers and clinicians are showing that boswella is indeed potent for inflammatory diseases such as arthritis. It effectively shrinks inflamed tissue, the underlying cause of pain, by improving the blood supply to the affected area and enhancing the repair of local blood vessels damaged by proliferating inflammation. This ability is attributed to chemical compounds in the gummy extract, scientifically known as boswellic acids. It is now an approved herbal medicine in India for use against osteoarthritis, rheumatoid arthritis, soft tissue rheumatism, low back pain, myositis and fibrositis.

TRADITIONAL AND OTHER THERAPEUTIC USES

- osteoarthritis and rheumatoid arthritis,
- soft tissue rheumatism, low back pain, myositis and fibrositis

TOXICITY, CAUTIONS AND CONTRAINDICATIONS

Experimental and clinical usage of boswella indicates it has none of the side effects on blood pressure, heart rate, or the gastric irritation and ulcers associated with many anti-inflammatory and antiarthritic drugs.

BURDOCK ROOT
(Arctium lappa)

ORIGIN
Africa, Europe, Asia

PART OF PLANT USED
Root

DESCRIPTION
Burdock is native to Africa and Europe, where its root has been used to improve immunity and overall health for at least 3,000 years. The plant produces a burr that gets stuck on people's clothing, and thus has been carried to every continent. In recent years, the burdock has come to be considered a weed, despised by lawn owners for its tenacious growth habits. The plant is a biennial, which means that in its second year it blooms and then dies. Burdock spends its first year of life working industriously to store all the necessary elements to bloom the following year. The part of the plant used in clearing the skin is the root, which is harvested in the autumn of the first year when its leaves begin to fall.

Burdock is excellent for any skin problems such as eczema, dandruff, non-healing wounds, infections that result in skin eruptions such as chicken pox, and common acne. Since acne is caused by infection in the skin's sebaceous glands, the herbal approach to fighting it is to strengthen the immune system. The root contains lignans including arctigenin, the glycosides arctiin and matairesinol, and polyacetylenes including tridecadienetetraynes, tridecatrienetriynes and a sulfur-containing arctic acid. It also contains amino acids including alpha guanidino-n-butyric acid, inulin, organic acids, fatty acids, and phenolic acids.

Burdock root tea must be taken three times a day for three to six months before one can expect to notice a significant improvement in skin condition. Fortunately, burdock tea is also generally beneficial to the constitution so that one can expect to enjoy better overall health in the process.

TRADITIONAL AND OTHER THERAPEUTIC USES

- gently stimulates health and the appearance of the skin
- improves the digestion and absorption of food
- cleanses the body by a stimulatory effect on the excretory systems, helping rid the body of toxins
- speeds the healing of the skin
- treats psoriasis, dandruff, wounds, ulcers, eczema, eruptions on the skin, boils, carbuncles, sties, sores, aphthous ulcerations and chronic acne
- taken internally, complements external application of calendula

CALENDULA
(Calendula officinalis)

ORIGIN
Unknown, possibly Mediterranean

PARTS OF PLANT USED
Flowers, stem and roots (extracted in water and alcohol)

DESCRIPTION
Calendula is a common garden plant that is as attractive as it is easy to grow. Its scientific name, Calendula officinalis, hints at what ancient physicians felt about its powers to heal and maintain skin in perfect health. Calendula is truly the miracle worker of the skin, whether a person has lumps or bumps, scabs that will not heal, eczema, athlete's foot, acne, or even herpes sores. Perusing old herbals, the reader quickly discovers that calendula has been used to treat virtually every skin condition. It is an all-purpose skin-healing agent. Not surprisingly, wherever calendula grows, it is used to treat the skin.

Calendula is commonly known as "pot marigold," "garden marigold," or sometimes just plain "marigold." This results in some confusion. There are two different and unrelated marigolds sold at garden centers: one, Calendula officinalis, is medicinal; the other, Tagetes erecta, is not. For this reason, particularly when talking about medicinal herbs, it is important to know and use the scientific name when discussing plants.

Calendula is a member of the Composite family, along with chrysanthemums, sunflowers, Jerusalem artichokes, elecampane, asters, thistles, chamomile, dandelion, burdock, and globe artichokes. A number of members of this family, most notably chamomile, elecampane, dandelion, and burdock, are used to treat skin problems. It would seem that this family contains a set of chemicals that in some fashion speed skin healing, although the exact nature of these chemicals and their actions remains a mystery. What is no mystery is that around the globe different ethnic groups, from the Arabs to the indigenous people of the Americas, were all using a daisy relative to increase the health of skin long before the age of international communication. No doubt this is more than a mere coincidence.

Calendula has been in cultivation for so long that no one really knows where it originated. It can be a perennial plant or an annual plant depending on the severity of the winter it must endure. People living in climates with temperatures well below freezing for months on end will have to plant calendula as an annual, but in more moderate climates, calendula will keep on going year after year. This preference for mild winters hints that the plant may have originated somewhere around the Mediterranean basin where the winters are mild.

Despite much analysis and research, the exact chemicals in calendula, giving it skin healing qualities, have not been isolated. Among its constituents are volatile oil, bitter substances, carotenoid substances (lycopin, neolycopin, citroxathin, carotin, violaxanthin, flavoxaanthin, chrysanthemaxanthin), gums, mucilage, resin, albumine, malic acid, cholesterin esters of laurin, myristin, palmatin acids, vitamin C, arnidol and faradiol (dihydroxy alcohols), calendin, triterpendiols, parafine, cerylalcholhol, stimasterin, glycosides and glucosides.

TRADITIONAL AND OTHER THERAPEUTIC USES
- antibacterial, , antiviral, antiprotozoal, and immunostimulatory
- antifungal that soothes itching of athlete's foot
- anti-inflammatory

- helps periodontal disease
- heals many ulcers in the mouth (e.g. herpetic)
- promotes re-epithelization (ability of broken or abraded skin to "heal over")
- applied as cream, reduces skin inflammation and itching of eczema
- flowers traditionally used in treatment of small pox and measles, as well as animal and insect bites

CASCARA SAGRADA
(Rhamnus purshiana)

ORIGIN
Pacific Northwest region of the United States

PART OF PLANT USED
Dried bark

DESCRIPTION
Cascara sagrada, "sacred bark" in Spanish, is a deciduous shrub or small tree from the buckhorn family with a distinctive reddish gray bark. The name dates back to the 17th century when the Native Americans introduced the Spanish and Mexican explorers to the usefulness of the bark for constipation and stomach upset. The bark was first marketed to the medical community in 1877 as a bitter emetic extract in liquid form. In 1890 the plant was officially listed in the U. S. Pharmacopoea.

Free anthraquinone and its sugar derivative, hydroxyanthracene derivative (HAD), are the active ingredients responsible for the laxative effect. These active substances cause increased peristalsis locally in the large intestine and also act at a distance by circulating in the bloodstream and stimulating a nerve center to trigger the laxative effect.

Cascara is perhaps the safest and most certain laxative available and can be used to restore tone to the colon and thereby overcome laxative dependence in the elderly. The herb is safe and effective for detoxifying and cleansing programs, as opposed to harsher laxatives, such as senna. Cascara is also an effective liver tonic in small doses. Cascara can be used as an effective chelating agent to prevent the occurrence of calcium-based urinary stones.

TRADITIONAL AND OTHER THERAPEUTIC USES

- laxative, cathartic, and purgative
- liver tonic
- cholagogue
- antibacterial agent
- chelating agent

TOXICITY, CAUTIONS AND CONTRAINDICATIONS

Cascara has no known toxicity at 50-100 mg. It takes from six to eight hours to produce its laxative effect. A cathartic effect can occur at very high doses. Cascara should not be used by nursing mothers since the laxative effect can be transmitted to their infants. It should not be used by people suffering from ulcers or irritable bowel syndrome.

CAT'S CLAW
(Uncaria tomentosa)

ORIGIN
Highlands of the Peruvian Amazon

PART OF PLANT USED
Bark (Roots are traditional and effective, but harvesting them kills the plant.)

DESCRIPTION
Uncaria tomentosa is commonly known in Spanish as una de gato and in English as "cat's claw." It is a giant, woody vine that grows more than 100 feet tall and is found wrapped around the trees in the highland rainforests of Peru. It is a slow growing vine taking 20 or more years to reach maturity, and is called cat's claw because the thorns found on the vine closely resemble the claws of a cat.

Historically, una de gato was used by natives as a tribal medicine for arthritis, gastritis, cancer and other diseases. The Peruvian Indians regard Uncaria tomentosa as a sacred herbal panacea, and their folklore suggests that una de gato has been successfully used in curing tumors and other known deadly diseases. The bark and roots have been used for hundreds and perhaps thousands of years by the native Ashanica Indians for treatment of a wide variety of health problems associated with the immune and digestive systems.

TRADITIONAL AND OTHER THERAPEUTIC USES
- improves allergic disorders
- treats dermatological disorders
- treats chronic inflammatory conditions such as arthritis, bursitis, and rheumatism
- may be beneficial in treating cancer, genital herpes

and herpes zoster, systemic candidiasis, diabetes, lupus, chronic fatigue syndrome, PMS and irregular female cycles, environmental toxin poisoning, and depression

- cleanses the entire intestinal tract and helps those suffering from a variety of stomach and bowel disorders including Crohn's disease, ulcers, gastritis, parasites, diverticulitis, hemorrhoids, leaky bowel syndrome and intestinal flora imbalance
- reduces side effects of AZT in AIDS treatment and radiation therapy for cancer
- reduces risk of heart attack by lowering blood pressure, increasing circulation and inhibiting the formation of plaques on the arterial walls
- reduces formation of blood clots in the vessels of the brain, heart and arteries

TOXICITY, CAUTIONS AND CONTRAINDICATIONS

Uncaria tomentosa is contraindicated for transplant recepients because of possible graft rejection. During pregnancy, or if nursing, una de gato should not be used. Diarrhea can occur in some cases.

European studies have determined that Uncaria tomentosa has very low toxicity even if taken in large amounts.

CHAMOMILE
(Matricaria recutita)

ORIGIN
Europe

DESCRIPTION
Chamomile, Matricaria recutita, is a member of the daisy family and is indigenous to Europe. It is not to be confused with Roman chamomile, Anthemis nobilis, an entirely different plant with a different medicinal action, used in shampoos and cosmetics. When in doubt, look to the Latin name.

A quick perusal through the literature of herbal medicine will show that chamomile, which grows wild from North Africa to Germany and west into Russia, has stood the test of time. People have collected the herb from the wild or bought it from the herb seller for more than 2,000 years, and used it to treat digestive ills including ulcers, upset stomachs, nausea, gas, constipation, diarrhea, and hemorrhoids.

Chamomile is just one member of the daisy family used in herbal medicine; others include elecampane, calendula, Echinacea, aster, Jerusalem artichoke, milk thistle and blessed thistle. All produce oils that are thought to be responsible for the medicinal actions. In clinical trials, the essential oils in chamomile have been proven to have anti-inflammatory, antispasmodic, antimicrobial and antiulcerative actions. Like other medicinal plants, it contains a complex series of chemicals that work individually and collectively on the body.

When your stomach hurts, the tissue lining your stomach is often irritated. Chamomile works to soothe irritated stomach tissue on two levels. One chemical contained in the plant is A-bisobol, which acts as an antiulcerative by speeding the mending of the torn tissues. A second chemical, chamazulene, acts as an anti-inflammatory. The problem with stomach linings is that they are filled with nerve endings, and when irritated stomach linings swell, it causes pressure on these nerves, which is experienced as pain. Chamazulene has the ability to shrink these tissues, relieving the pressure on the nerves. Thus, the first chemical heals the tissue, thus ending the source of inflammation, and another treats the inflammation itself. These are just two of the chemicals found in chamomile!

TRADITIONAL AND OTHER THERAPEUTIC USES

- treats nausea and digestive disorders
- antimicrobial action; one ingredient, azulene, can kill both Staphylococcus and Streptococcus infections
- strengthens "delicate" gastrointestinal tract
- soothes nerves, acting as a mild sedative
- stimulates production of digestive juices

CINNAMON
(Cinnamonum zeylanicum), (C. cassis)

ORIGIN
Primarily Sri Lanka

PART OF PLANT USED
Dried inner bark

DESCRIPTION
Cinnamon is an ancient spice made from the highly aromatic reddish or yellow-brown bark of several trees of the genus Cinnamonum. Cinnamon trees are relatively small, about 30 feet in height. They have stiff oblong evergreen leaves and silky clusters of yellowish white flowers with dry pointed fruit. Before harvesting, the stems are slit on each side. The outer corky bark is pulled off and the aromatic inner portions are scraped and dried into "quills" and baled for export. The extracted cinnamon oil is used as a flavoring and pharmacologic ingredient for medicinals, particularly mouthwashes. The finest quality cinnamon comes from the Cinnamonum zeylanicum of Sri Lanka. Cinnamonum evergreens of the Lauraceae family grow in Java, the West Indies, Brazil, and Egypt. They have even been grown in limited number in California and south Florida.

Cinnamon oil has many uses today. It is a favorite flavor for many mouthwash preparations. In some systems of medicine in this world, cinnamon is thought to be an invigorator. It has also been regarded as a detoxicant. Since cinnamon promotes perspiration and increased metabolism, it would naturally be a good candidate for cleansing. Cinnamon is also a very powerful astringent with strong antiseptic activity. Not only does cinnamon refresh the mouth, but its antimicrobial action may also be useful in combating the spread of plaque-forming bacteria.

One of the most esoteric attributes of cinnamon may be its ability to affect levels of specific hormones. There are many plant extracts that have been known to affect the levels of certain hormones; for example, brewer's yeast can potentiate insulin. In a similar manner, cinnamon has been shown to stimulate the utilization of glucose in the presence of insulin. Other spices known to have similar insulin-like effects are turmeric, bay leaves and cloves. Although scientists still do not know completely what is the mechanism for the insulin-like activity of cinnamon, it is thought to interact with serum albumin to achieve its effect. It is postulated that the active component of cinnamon probably binds to albumin, resulting in a new complex that potentiates the activity. The exact chemical term that reflects cellular changes is "glucose oxidation." Cinnamon stimulates glucose oxidation and may be useful therapeutically for people with abnormal sugar metabolism. By having a positive effect on serum glucose levels, overall body conditions are better for the growth of probiotic bacteria. This results in less dependency on alcoholic mouthwashes.

In May of 1995, a study was done by the Japanese to assess the superoxide dismutase-like activity of natural antioxidants. Superoxide dismutase (SOD) is widely recognized as one of the body's main antioxidant enzymes. In that study, a variety of natural antioxidants were tested for their free radical scavenging ability. Among the substances measured were vitamin C, glutathione, catechins and epitcatechins (found in green teas). These natural antioxidants are water-soluble antioxidants. Cinnamon, however, is a lipophilic (fat-soluble) antioxidant. Other lipophilic antioxidants were also tested, such as gamma oryzanol, rosemary leaf, alpha-lecithin, and alpha-cephalin. The results of this study indicated that cinnamon contains oils which have SOD-like activity.

Today, we can find cinnamon utilized in non-food applications, such lip sunscreen, toothpaste, mouthwashes and chewing gum. These definitely make sense when we consider that cinnamon has astringent and antimicrobial characteristics. Basically, not only will it freshen your mouth, but it may also inhibit the spread of pathogenic bacteria on the lips, tongue and oral cavity.

TRADITIONAL AND OTHER THERAPEUTIC USES

- stimulates glucose utilization in the presence of insulin
- stimulates glucose oxidation and sugar metabolism
- acts as a lipophilic antioxidant
- useful as an astringent and oral antiseptic

TOXICITY, CAUTIONS AND CONTRAINDICATIONS

Cinnamon is considered safe when used in moderation.

CLOVE
(Syzygium aromaticum)

ORIGIN
West Indies, Indonesia, India, Sri Lanka

PART OF PLANT USED
Flower bud

DESCRIPTION
Clove oil is obtained from the distillation of small flower buds of the tropical evergreen tree, Syzygium aromaticum. Also known as Eugenia caryophyllata, it is native to Madagascar and to the Indonesian island of Moluccas. Clove trees grow to a height of 25 to 40 feet (eight to 12 m) and each can produce up to 75 pounds (34 kg) of dried buds. The abundant clusters of small, red flower buds are harvested just before blooming and are dried. They become hard, brown, and peg-like in appearance.

Used in cooking, soaps, perfumes, and natural mouthwashes, clove's flavor is pungent with menthol-type aftertaste. Typically, it is combined with ylang ylang, ginger, vanilla, cinnamon, tea tree oil, peppermint and bay leaf. The main active ingredient in clove oil is eugenol. In addition to antibacterial effects, it is a powerful topical anesthetic. These two very important qualities make clove oil an ideal mouthwash ingredient.

Although approved by the American Dental Association as an anesthetic, clove has many other potential uses, which have not yet been scrutinized by the Western scientific community. As a result, anyone who looks for information on cloves may have a difficult time finding good, hard research regarding its qualities. However, it has been a recognized asset in many of the different medicinal systems around the world, particularly Asia.

TRADITIONAL AND OTHER THERAPEUTIC USES

- kills mouth odors when used in mouthwash and/or toothpaste
- analgesic, as in tooth ache, and antineuralgic
- antispasmodic action on muscles reducing inflammation and cramps
- antiseptic with antifungal and anti-parasitic properties (e.g. ringworm)
- reportedly effective as an aphrodisiac and may help with premature ejaculation problems
- expectorant, useful in coughs and colds
- mild stimulant action, helping combat fatigue
- digestive aid
- elevates low blood pressure

TOXICITY, CAUTIONS AND CONTRAINDICATIONS

Do not use if hypertensive or if pregnant. It may irritate the skin with topical use.

DAMIANA

PART OF PLANT USED
Leaves and flower buds

DESCRIPTION

There are herbal medicines that combat the effect of stress on our bodies, physically, mentally, and emotionally. If your "nerves" are taking a beating, you might want to think about taking a daily tonic to strengthen and nourish them. The herb damiana is used to generally strengthen the nervous system, especially with respect to stress. Damiana can be found growing throughout the southern United States, Mexico, and well into Central American. It looks much like oregano. The whole stems are harvested when the plants bloom. Once they are dried, they are stripped of their leaves and buds, which are the parts used in herbal preparations.

Damiana is used as a commercial flavoring. It is used as an ingredient in alcoholic and non-alcoholic beverages, frozen dairy desserts, candy, baked goods, gelatins, and puddings. The plant is rated by the U.S. Food and Drug Administration as being food safe.

The native people of northern Mexico have long collected the plant from the wild to treat nervous and muscular debility, especially when this is due to overexertion. In Latin America, the indiginous people used damiana as a treatment for bed-wetting in children. This problem has now been established to be a functional condition related to stress, and it comes as no surprise that there is an increase in bed-wetting as the summer draws to a close and children begin to anticipate their return to school.

Western physicians discovered that damiana acts to strengthen the nervous system, particularly when the patient has been pushed to the brink of nervous exhaustion.

Damiana counters weakness by gently building up the system, not by acting as a stimulant such as caffeine. One of the Eclectics, Dr. Finley Ellingwood, said of damiana, "Dr. Reid uses damiana in all conditions where a general tonic is needed, especially if there be enfeeblement of the central nervous system. He esteems it most highly, prescribing it constantly for this purpose." If you ever experience "enfeeblement" at the end of the day, damiana can be helpful in its capacity as a gentle, general tonic.

Damiana contains volatile oils including thymol, b-cadinene, calamene, cineole, pinene, and calamenene; and also flavonoids, hydroquinones, cyanogenetic glycoside, damianin, resin, and tannins. Which chemicals or combinations impact the nervous system remains a mystery.

Damiana has been long known as an aphrodisiac. It is unclear whether this impact is due to the strengthening effect damiana has on the nervous system, which in turn normalizes sexual desire, or whether it contains chemicals that fire up the libido. Interestingly, in Latin America, a liqueur is made out of damiana that is called by the same name. Eclectic physician Finley Ellingwood from earlier this century had this to say about this aspect of the herb, "A mild nerve tonic claimed to be caluave in the treatment of sexual impotence. Some of our physicians praise it highly for its influence in sexual neurasthenia, and it is said to correct frigidity in the female. It had long enjoyed a local reputation as a stimulant tonic of the sexual apparatus among the natives of Mexico, before it attracted the attention of the profession. Besides its peculiar action on the sexual appetite and function, it is a general tonic, somewhat cathartic and is slightly cholagogue. The midwives and women of loose morals of western Mexico also attribute emmenagogue properties to it."

The Eclectics felt that damiana both steadied the nerves and stimulated the general constitution to improve health. If mental exhaustion is masquerading as depression, adding Damiana to one's daily health regime may be appropriate. The plant is safe and suited to long-term use. Like other herbal tonics, it takes a while to work on the "nerves," and maybe a few weeks before its effects are noted.

TRADITIONAL AND OTHER THERAPEUTIC USES
- nerve tonic
- aphrodisiac

TOXICITY, CAUTIONS AND CONTRADICTION
None noted.

DANDELION
(Taraxacum officinale)

PARTS OF PLANT USED
Leaves and root

DESCRIPTION
Dandelion is one of the best herbs for cleansing and strengthening the liver, even helping hepatitis, jaundice and cirrhosis. There are claims that dandelion can effectively heal hepatitis when six cups of tea from the raw root are taken each day for a week or two. It stimulates the secretion of bile, thus aiding digestion, acting as a laxative and breaking up gall and kidney stones. Its blood cleansing properties also can cause improvement in skin rashes, measles, chicken pox, eczema, poison oak and ivy and other skin eruptions. The Chinese use it for infections, inflammations, boils, abscesses, swellings, carious teeth, red swollen and painful eyes, and fever and other heat-related conditions. Externally, its juice is applied to snake bites.

Dandelion's action on the digestive system is also notable. It stimulates and strengthens the digestive process and is valuable for diabetics and hypoglycemics. It is useful for detoxification from overeating meat and fatty and fried foods. Its diuretic effect cleanses the kidneys and lowers blood pressure. For the breasts, dandelion may help reduce sores, tumors, swollen lymph nodes and cysts, and possibly help prevent some forms of breast cancer. It also stimulates the production of breast milk. Dandelion leaf tea taken cool is one of the most effective diuretics.

The leaves are very high in iron, vitamins and minerals, especially vitamin A and potassium, and are useful for treating anemia. Eaten when young in the spring, they help clear out any excesses from winter, aiding in the prevention of spring colds. The root can be roasted and made into a strong tea, which Europeans call "dandelion coffee." It actually is an excellent coffee substitute, since its full-bodied, bitter flavor is satisfying and counteracts the effects of previous caffeine by cleansing the liver. It combines well with chicory and burdock roots for a closer coffee flavor. In general, the roasted roots can be used by those suffering from "coldness," and the uncooked roots by those with "heat."

Active constituents include an acrid bitter resin (taraxacerin), inulin (25 percent), phytosterols, saponins, glutin, gum potash, and vitamins A and C (the vitamin A content is higher than in carrots). It is a bitter tonic, diuretic, lithotriptic, astringent, cholagogue, galactogogue, laxative and alterative.

TRADITIONAL AND OTHER THERAPEUTIC USES
- indigestion and constipation
- liver congestion, hepatitis, jaundice, and cirrhosis
- skin eruptions
- breast sores
- tumors and cysts
- promotion of lactation
- urinary bladder and kidney infections
- kidney stones and gallstones
- diabetes and hypoglycemia

DEVIL'S CLAW
(Harpogophytum procumbens)

ORIGIN
Africa, particularly southern Africa

PART OF PLANT USED
Fruit

DESCRIPTION
Devil's claw derives its name from its large hooked, claw-like fruit, which has been known to harm and trap livestock grazing nearby. The tuber is used medicinally and has become a primary treatment for arthritis and rheumatism. In Africa the root is also used as a treatment for indigestion and other gastrointestinal problems in the same manner as Western bitters are used. Devil's claw also possesses a bitter value of 6,000, equivalent to gentian root, the main western bitter.

It is also used to treat skin rashes, wounds, etc. Two components of the plant, harpogoside and beta sitosterol have anti-inflammatory properties. Whole devil's claw, however, was found to be superior to isolated harpogoside.

The British Herbal Pharmacopoea recognizes devil's claw as having anti-inflammatory, antirheumatic, analgesic, sedative and diuretic properties. In addition, it has proved effective in treating such complaints as dyspepsia and conditions relating to the proper functioning of bile salts, the gall bladder, and the enterohepatic circuit.

TRADITIONAL AND OTHER THERAPEUTIC USES
- anti-inflammatory properties helpful for sufferers of arthritis and inflammatory diseases
- treat liver, gall bladder and kidney ailments
- reduce lymphatic system toxicity

- diabetes
- nervous malaise
- respiratory ailments
- blood diseases
- indigestion.

TOXICITY, CAUTIONS AND CONTRAINDICATIONS

Devil's claw has extremely low toxicity and side effects are rare. Its use should be avoided during pregnancy as it has been suggested that it stimulates uterine muscle.

DONG QUAI (DANG KWEI)
(Angelica sinensis)

ORIGIN
Asia, primarily China, Korea, Japan

PART OF PLANT USED
Dried root

DESCRIPTION
Chinese angelica root, dong quai (or dang kwei - rhyming with "wrong way") is the most important female tonic remedy in Chinese medicine. It is used for debility and poor vitality, convalescence and fatigue in women as well as all kinds of gynecological, menstrual, or menopausal symptoms. Dong quai is the Chinese name of the root of the plant, Angelica sinensis, belonging to the family, Umbelliferaceae. It is related to the European angelica, but its medicinal actions are more potent. The plant is a tall umbelliferous plant with branched celery-like leaves and a tall umbel of white-green flowers.

Ligustilide, butylene phthalide and butyl phthalide are found in the volatile aromatic oil while ferulic acid and various polysaccharides are found in the non-aromatic fractions. Dong quai has an immediate and stimulating effect on the uterus, especially during pregnancy or delivery. It has been clinically observed to strengthen and normalize uterine contractions. These effects are thought to be due to components of the volatile oil, particularly ligustilide. Symptoms such as menstrual pain and irregularities, recurrent spontaneous abortion, chills in the hands and feet, anemia and in some cases, sterility, have also responded well to dong quai. Animal and human studies have shown that dong quai also improves peripheral circulation and reduces blood viscosity. Research suggests that both ferulic acid and ligustilide are responsible for preventing spasms, relaxing vessels, and reducing blood clotting in peripheral vessels.

TRADITIONAL AND OTHER THERAPEUTIC USES

- the main female tonic in Asia (ginseng has been the more traditional male tonic)
- provides energy, vitality, and resistance to disease
- regulates female hormones
- treats most menstrual and menopausal problems
- beneficial in pregnancy and delivery
- blood tonic, promoting its production and circulation
- used in treating anemia, boils, headache, and venous problems, including peripheral blood flow

TOXICITY, CAUTIONS AND CONTRAINDICATIONS

Side effects to dong quai are extremely rare. Rare cases of pyrogenia have been reported, but required no treatment. People with gastrointestinal disease may experience diarrhea. Dong quai should be avoided in those with hemorrhagic disease, hypermenorrhea, during at least the first three months of pregnancy, and during severe flu.

ECHINACEA
(Echinacea purpurea, E. angustifolia, E. pallida)

ORIGIN
North America, cultivated in Europe

PARTS OF PLANT USED
Root/rhizome

DESCRIPTION
Echinacea was the remedy the Native Americans from the Plains region used for wounds, infections, and insect and snake bites. The purple coneflower is a member of the sunflower family. Echinacea is a two- to five-foot perennial plant whose purple flowers are similar to the black-eyed Susan daisy. Echinacea is probably the most popular American immune-enhancing herb available today. It is well known for its strong antibiotic-like effects and is very useful for a variety of ailments including fevers, boils, wounds, tonsillitis, bronchitis, respiratory infections, and eczema. Echinacea kills a broad range of viruses, bacteria and fungi. Echinacoside, a natural antibiotic-like alkaloid, improves the body's own resistance to infectious conditions. Echinacea also strengthens tissues against bacterial and viral assault. The three most common species are Echinacea angustifolia, E. purpurea, and E. pallida. In the United States, the roots of E. angustifolia have been used traditionally. Europe has performed more studies with fresh plant extracts of E. purpurea.

Echinacea is rich in polysaccharides and phytosterols, which have potent non-specific stimulatory actions on the immune system. Research has indicated that they stimulate the "alternative complement" pathway which helps activate general immune cells to scavenge for bacteria and cellular debris. The roots of E. angustifolia contain significant amounts of glycoside echinacoside. Echinacoside has mild antibiotic activity. Other components in Echinacea, such as the polysaccharide echinacin, also have antibiotic and antifungal activity. E. purpurea contains components with cortisone-like activity, which help with wound healing by inhibiting inflammatory hyaluronidase enzyme. E. purpurea also contains the sesquiterpene esters which have immunostimulatory activity.

Echinacea has been used to boost the immune system, to help speed wound healing, to reduce inflammations, and to treat colds, flu and infections. Many of the active components of Echinacea have antibacterial, antiviral, and antifungal properties. Echinacea has also been used externally to cleanse and heal wounds, eczema, burns, psoriasis, herpes, vaginitis, canker sores, abscesses, and other skin conditions. Recent research has indicated that Echinacea has potent anti-tumor activity and helps stimulate the immune system to destroy cancer cells.

TRADITIONAL AND OTHER THERAPEUTIC USES

- immune stimulator, helpful with colds and influenza, infections of the eyes, ears, and urinary tract, strept throat, tonsillitis, inflamed gums, and wound healing and cleansing (ulcerations and sores)
- anti-inflammatory, analgesic, sedative, and anti-spasmodic
- pain and swelling in inflammation and water retention
- possible anticancer agent
- treat snake and insect bites
- treat boils, abscesses, gangrene
- treat urticaria (external wash) and for other allergy relief

TOXICITY, CAUTIONS AND CONTRAINDICATIONS

There is no reported toxicity. Side effects from Echinacea are rare. Persons with kidney disorders should restrict usage to 10 days of intake due to possible imbalance in excreted minerals.

EPHEDRA
(Ephedra sinica, E. girardiana, E. equisatina, E. dystachia)

ORIGIN
China, India, Middle East

PARTS OF PLANT USED
Stems and leaves (above-ground parts)

DESCRIPTION
Ephedra, or ma huang, is a perennial herb belonging to the gymnosperms. The plant is made up of slender aerial green stems with small vestigial leaves. Ephedra has been used in Chinese medicine for thousands of years for bronchial spasms and as a stimulant for the sympathetic nervous system.

Ephedra is a source of ephedrine, an alkaloid similar to adrenaline in its ability to excite the sympathetic nervous system. Ephedrine was used earlier in the century as a cure for asthma since it relaxes airways. But the isolated drug fell into disfavor when it was found to raise blood pressure. The whole plant however contains a mixture of alkaloids, which counteract the activities of ephedrine, resulting in a safer and more balanced action. Ephedradines and pseudo-ephedrine lower blood pressure and reduce heart rate while still relaxing smooth muscle and opening the respiratory system.

Ephedra has been used in China and Europe to treat asthma, hay fever, allergies, arthritis and fevers, clear blocked sinuses, raise blood pressure and increase alertness and perception. Ephedra is a stimulant of the sympathetic nervous system, which controls the "fight or flight" response of the body.

TRADITIONAL AND OTHER THERAPEUTIC USES

- bronchodilator (has been used for asthma, bronchitis, and catarrh in the upper respiratory tract)
- circulatory system stimulant
- appetite reducer
- diuretic
- anti-allergenic
- reduces cough, nasal congestion, chills and "cold" fevers
- treats urticaria
- treats enuresis
- treats hypotension

TOXICITY, CAUTIONS & CONTRAINDICATIONS

Ephedra has been banned by the U.S. Food and Drug Administration. Ephedra is contraindicated with high or even moderately elevated blood pressure. It should not be taken together with other CNS stimulants or circulatory agents (e.g. digitoxin or beta-blockers).

Please note that ephedra can be dangerous in high dosages, and a single high dose could result in irregular heartbeats. Use moderately and with caution.

EVENING PRIMROSE OIL
(Oenothera biennis)

ORIGIN
North America

PART OF PLANT USED
Oil from seeds

DESCRIPTION
Evening primrose is a large, delicate wild flower, which grows in North America from the Rocky Mountains to the Atlantic seaboard. It can reach up to eight feet tall and is seen along streams and roads in the high desert at altitudes up to 9,000 feet. The flowers bloom in the evening, pollinated by night-flying insects.

The value of evening primrose lies in the gamma-linolenic acid (GLA) content of its oil. GLA is an important intermediary in the metabolic conversion of linoleic acid to prostaglandin E1. The normal diet is quite sufficient in the essential fatty acid linoleic acid (LA), but the first step in its conversion to prostaglandin E1 can be easily blocked. Among the known blocking agents are viruses, carcinogens, cholesterol, saturated fatty acids, trans fatty acids, alcohol, insufficient insulin, excess dietary alpha-linolenic acid (ALA) (found in linseed and black currant oils), radiation, and the aging process. Traditional dietary GLA can therefore be extremely valuable since it skips this potential blockage and provides a material from which prostaglandin E1 can easily be produced.

TRADITIONAL AND OTHER THERAPEUTIC USES

- relieve premenstrual syndrome (PMS) symptoms
- treats benign breast disease
- lowers high serum cholesterol
- treats atopic eczema
- possible treatment of psoriasis and rheumatoid arthritis when used in combination with fish oils
- encouraging results with multiple sclerosis sufferers
- makes withdrawal from alcohol intake easier and can relieve post-drinking depression
- possibly useful in treatment of schizophrenia, heart disease and obesity

TOXICITY, CAUTIONS & CONTRAINDICATIONS

Evening primrose oil has very low toxicity and has been used without harm at levels of up to 5-6 g daily. Occasionally, evening primrose oil may cause nausea, headaches or skin eruptions when first taken. This symptom quickly subsides over a period of time and can be lessened by taking the dosage with a meal.

Evening primrose oil should be avoided by epileptics as it may exacerbate a certain type of temporal lobe epilepsy.

Also, evening primrose oil is best not taken with the drugs methotrimeprazine and procarbazine, both of which depress the central nervous system. Evening primrose oil should be avoided by those taking blood-thinning drugs, such as warfarin.

EYEBRIGHT
(Euphrasia officinalis)

ORIGIN
Britain, common in temperate regions

PART OF PLANT USED
Extract, principally of flowers

DESCRIPTION
Common "eyebright" is a small, low herb, usually with one blackish green stalk rising up. From the bottom, it spreads into sundry branches, whereon are small and almost round, yet pointed, dark green leaves, two always set together. It has small white flowers, steeped with purple and yellow spots, or stripes. These develop into small round heads with very small seeds therein. Eyebright grows in meadows and grassy places in North America. It flowers in July.

Eyebright may be taken internally or made into eye drops. It has been used for many years to treat a variety of ailments affecting the eyes.

TRADITIONAL AND OTHER THERAPEUTIC USES
- helps all infirmities of the eyes that impair sight
- traditionally used to improve memory and brain function
- treats catarrhal inflammations of the eye

FENUGREEK

DESCRIPTION

Although originally from southeastern Europe and western Asia, fenugreek is now grown in many parts of the world, including India, northern Africa, and the United States. The seeds of fenugreek contain the most potent medicinal effects of the plant.

A number of uses were found for fenugreek in ancient times. Medicinally it was used for the treatment of wounds, abscesses, arthritis, bronchitis, and digestive problems. Traditional Chinese herbalists used it for kidney problems and conditions affecting the male reproductive tract. Fenugreek was, and remains, a food and a spice commonly eaten in many parts of the world. The steroidal saponins account for many of the beneficial effects of fenugreek, particularly the inhibition of cholesterol absorption and synthesis. The seeds are rich in dietary fiber, which may be the main reason it can lower blood sugar levels in diabetes.

Due to the somewhat bitter taste of fenugreek seeds, debitterized seeds or encapsulated products are preferred. The typical range of intake is 5-30 grams with each meal or 15-90 grams all at once with one meal. As a tincture, fenugreek can be taken up to three times per day.

TRADITIONAL AND OTHER THERAPEUTIC USES
- constipation
- diabetes
- high cholesterol
- high triglycerides

TOXICITY, CAUTIONS AND CONTRAINDICATIONS

Use of more than 100 grams of fenugreek seeds daily can cause intestinal upset and nausea. Otherwise, fenugreek is extremely safe.

FEVERFEW
(Tanacetum parthenium)

ORIGIN
Germany, Netherlands, Great Britain, Israel

PART OF PLANT USED
Leaves

DESCRIPTION

Feverfew is a member of the daisy family, similar to chrysanthemum. The herb has become popular with recent clinical trials showing its effectiveness as a remedy for migraine headaches. It was known to the ancient Egyptians and Greeks as a valuable herbal remedy, used as an anti-inflammatory agent, to treat headaches, and as an emmenagogue (promoting menstrual flow).

Feverfew contains bitter-tasting sesquiterpene lactones of which parthenolide is the most pharmacologically active. Research studies determined that parthenolide, michefuscalide, and chrysanthenyl acetate inhibited the production of prostaglandin. This inhibition of prostaglandin results in reduction in inflammation, decreased secretion of histamine, decreased activation of inflammatory cells and a reduction of fever, from where the name of the herb derives. This reduction of prostaglandins and histamine is thought to be part of the reason for the efficacy of feverfew in treating migraine headaches by reducing spasm of blood vessels.

With its anti-inflammatory activities, feverfew has also been useful against swelling in arthritis. It has been used for relaxing the smooth muscles in the uterus, promoting menstrual flow; and inhibiting platelet aggregation and excessive blood clotting. As a bitter herb, feverfew has also been useful in stimulating digestion and improving the functioning of the liver.

TRADITIONAL AND OTHER THERAPEUTIC USES

- treats inflammation of arthritis, "hot" swellings, and acute fever
- treats migraine and tension headaches
- alleviates nausea and vomiting and is used as a digestive aid
- vertigo
- as an emmenagogue in those with menstrual difficulties
- depression
- asthma
- as a liver tonic
- as a sleep aid

TOXICITY, CAUTIONS AND CONTRAINDICATIONS

No toxicity has been seen in clinical trials.

GARCINIA
(Garcinia cambogia)

ORIGIN
India (Western Ghats)

PART OF PLANT USED
Rind of fruit

DESCRIPTION
One researcher tried the Garcinia fruit and said that "as little as one gram before each meal was extremely effective in reducing my own appetite and weight and resulted in a definite sustained increase in energy and a weight loss for me of about one pound per day without any dieting. However, my results may not be typical."

Research has been done on the effects of the purified active ingredient, (-)-HCA, in its sodium salt form, which has been found to be considerably more powerful than the crude powder and has important additional functions. (-)-HCA has been shown in animal experiments to suppress both appetite and the formation of fats and cholesterol in the liver. In addition, it results in an increase in LDL receptor activity in liver cells that can pull LDL cholesterol out of circulation. If further research shows that other mechanisms do not increase LDL production enough to compensate, then (-)-HCA is likely to be adopted as a cholesterol-lowering agent. There is no reduction in protein or muscle tissue to detract from the reduction of circulating fatty acids and total lipid levels in the body. Furthermore, there is an increase in glycogen production that may be the cause of the perceived energy increase mentioned above. Finally, (-)-HCA does not speed up metabolism or produce the side effects of amphetamines, and does not create strong aversions to foods. In animal studies, (-)-HCA retained its full effectiveness in reducing food intake for one month of sustained use, and for 80 days of interrupted use.

It is uncertain how (-)-HCA reduces appetite. Possibilities include feedback controls tied to glycogen and glucose levels in the liver (glucose sensitive fibers have been found in the vagus nerve within the liver). In experiments with carbon-14-labeled (-)-HCA, C-14 was found in the brain and in the hypothalamus, the seat of appetite regulation. A mechanism of action in the hypothalamus has not yet been established. Studies show that (-)-HCA reduces fatty acid and cholesterol production in the liver by inhibiting the citrate cleavage enzyme (ATP: citrate oxaloacetate lyase). This enzyme is required to cleave excess citrate into oxaloacetate and acetyl-CoA. Acetyl-CoA is the source of two carbon units required for fatty acid and cholesterol biosynthesis outside the mitochondria. (-)-HCA does not act inside the mitochondria, therefore normal energy production in the Krebs', or citric acid, cycle is not interrupted. The decrease in carbon unit availability for cholesterol synthesis results in increased activity of low-density lipoprotein (LDL) receptors. The increased LDL-receptor activity results in significant increases in the amount of LDL cholesterol that is bound to the cells and degraded, reducing the LDL portion of the total body cholesterol.

GARLIC
(Allium sativa)

DESCRIPTION

Thousands of years of use, coupled with modern scientific research, have shown garlic to be an herb with important health properties. An Egyptian papyrus of around 1550 BCE includes 22 therapeutic recipes that use garlic for complaints ranging from bites to heart problems and tumors. The Greeks, Romans and Vikings have all left evidence that garlic was prescribed for a variety of illnesses.

Intact raw garlic cells contain alliin (an amino acid) and alliinase (an enzyme). When garlic is cut or crushed, alliin and alliinase immediately react together to produce the pungent substance allicin. Allicin kills all sorts of cells, including germs.

Traditional Chinese herbalists prescribed garlic cloves, aged for two to three years in vinegar, to help many complaints. Today, cold-aged garlic is in principle similar to this ancient remedy. Although raw garlic is actually an oxidant rather than an antioxidant; cold-aging process reverses this and turns garlic into a strong antioxidant.

TRADITIONAL AND OTHER THERAPEUTIC USES

- can help to decrease total cholesterol while increasing HDL ("good") cholesterol
- protects against free radicals and oxidation
- antifungal and antibacterial; effective in numerous health problems such as colds and influenza
- has been shown to boost the activity of the body's immune system, including natural killer cells
- can increase the speed of clearance of Candida albicans cells from the body
- suitable for use in catarrhal, respiratory or bronchial conditions

TOXICITY, CAUTIONS AND CONTRAINDICATIONS

Garlic has been tested extensively for toxicity, and no amount of it seems to cause harmful side effects. There are no known drug interactions or contraindications for garlic.

CHINESE GARLIC
(Allium sativum)

ORIGIN
China (Xianjiang province)

PART OF PLANT USED
Cloves

DESCRIPTION
Chinese garlic is a perennial plant with white, starry flowers and bulb clusters of individual cloves. It has been used for both culinary and medical purposes. The plant has been used to protect against infections, to lower blood cholesterol and fat levels, and to help with digestion. Modern research has confirmed these effects. The Chinese have valued garlic for thousands of years for its extraordinary healing properties and have recently discovered a unique and meticulous way to process the garlic cloves in order to stabilize the active ingredients and to maximize the Total Allicin Potential (TAP) that reaches the consumer.

The principle active agent in garlic is alliin. When garlic cloves are cut or bruised, the alliin is converted to the pungent-smelling allicin by the action of the enzyme allinase. Extreme care must be taken during processing of the cloves to maximize the TAP of garlic. Any bruising of the cloves or harsh treatment would result in conversion of the alliin to allicin and loss of the active ingredients. Alliin and allicin are sulfur-containing components. The sulfur compounds have antibiotic and antifungal effects. They help stop the liver from making too much cholesterol and reduce clotting tendencies.

TRADITIONAL AND OTHER THERAPEUTIC USES

- protects and fights against infections, colds and flu
- antibiotic, antifungal, antiviral, anti-Candidal, antiparasitic, and antiprotozoan
- expectorant, reduce phlegm, bronchitis, asthma, and pneumonia
- protects wounds from infection, treat abscesses, cuts
- protects the circulation, lowering cholesterol and fat levels
- "thins" the blood, reducing blood clotting (thrombosis)
- lowers blood sugar levels
- antitoxin (carcinogens, heavy metals, drugs, poisons)
- stimulates and protects the liver
- possibly anticarcinogenic
- digestive tonic, helpful in gastritis and dysentery

TOXICITY, CAUTIONS AND CONTRAINDICATIONS

No toxicity has been reported.

GINGER
(Zingiber officinale)

ORIGIN
Israel, China, India, Nigeria

PART OF PLANT USED
Rhizomes

DESCRIPTION

Ginger is one of the most widely used roots both for culinary purposes and for medicinal ones. Recent medical studies have confirmed the ancient uses of ginger as a carminative, cholalogue, antitussive, diaphoretic and to help the absorption of other remedies throughout the body.

The main components of ginger are the aromatic essential oil, antioxidants and the pungent oleoresin. The pungent compounds have been identified as the phenylalkylketones, known as gingerols, shogaols and zingerone.

Most of the medicinal effects of ginger appear to be due to the pungent components, which are standardized. Recent research published in The Lancet and other prestigious journals have confirmed the traditional uses for ginger. Ginger was found more effective than drugs at treating motion sickness and nausea. Ginger is able to calm the stomach, promote bile flow and improve the appetite. Ginger is also known for its warming expectorant action on the upper respiratory tract, suppressing coughs and encouraging the release of mucus and phlegm. With its diaphoretic action, promoting sweating and increasing circulation, it is additionally useful for colds and low grade fevers. Ginger tea has long been a standard remedy for sore throats, colds and flu. Recent studies have found that ginger lowers blood cholesterol and reduces blood clotting. The pungent compound, gingerol, has been found to have a structure similar to the well-known anticoagulant aspirin, which may explain the similar effect that the two compounds have on prostaglandin. Ginger is also a very effective antibiotic agent and strong antioxidant.

TRADITIONAL AND OTHER THERAPEUTIC USES

- nausea, vomiting, motion sickness, vertigo, and morning sickness
- increases appetite
- stomach ache, dyspepsia, flatulence, and indigestion
- promotes bile flow
- fights colds, coughs, influenza, and fever
- lowers high cholesterol
- antioxidant
- "thins" the blood

TOXICITY, CAUTIONS & CONTRAINDICATIONS

No toxicity.

GINKGO
(Ginkgo biloba)

ORIGIN
China, Japan, now grown worldwide

PART OF PLANT USED
Leaves

DESCRIPTION
Ginkgo biloba is one of the world's oldest living tree species, believed to have survived for 200 million years. Individual trees have lived 1,000 years. Ginkgo trees are tall and hardy, highly resistant to pollutants and pests, with distinctive fan-shaped bi-lobed leaves. Considered a sacred tree by the Chinese, it has been used since ancient times for respiratory ailments and for brain function. Hundreds of studies have been performed with Ginkgo biloba extracts confirming many of the ancient uses as well as finding new applications.

Gingko biloba extract has been shown in clinical studies to increase the rate at which information is transmitted at the nerve cell level. In a double blind clinical study, Ginkgo biloba extract was shown to produce restoration of vigilance to approximately normal levels together with improved mental performance in elderly patients. The conclusion of the study also indicated regular Ginkgo biloba use has a positive effect in geriatric subjects with regard to deterioration of mental performance. It may be of benefit in many cases of senility, including Alzheimer's disease.

The main active compounds in Ginkgo leaves are the flavoglycosides: kaempferol, quercetin, isorhamnetin, and proanthocyanidins. These compounds have antioxidant and anti-free radical properties. Also important are the terpenes: ginkgolides and bilobalides. One way these agents decrease inflammation is by inhibiting Platelet Activating Factor (PAF) and reducing the stickiness of platelets, which can otherwise result in decreased circulatory flow. High PAF has been implicated in a wide variety of diseases including asthma, heart arrhythmias, myocardial infarction and atherosclerosis.

TRADITIONAL AND OTHER THERAPEUTIC USES

- cerebrovascular insufficiency, vertigo, related headaches, tinnitis, and dizziness
- improves mental performance and brain function
- senility, memory loss, dementia, and possibly helpful in Alzheimer's disease
- peripheral vascular diseases, Raynaud's syndrome, and limb numbness and tingling
- migraine headaches
- ischemia
- hypoxia and asthma
- impotence and erectile dysfunction
- hemorrhoids
- inflammation
- allergies

TOXICITY, CAUTIONS AND CONTRAINDICATIONS

There has been no reported toxicity other than rare cases of gastric upset or headaches. Also, some have reported cases of intraocular bleeding when taken in combination with non-steroidal anti-inflammatory drugs (NSAID) such as ibuprofen. If blurry vision is experienced, discontinue use of the herb, the NSAID, or both.

GINSENG

DESCRIPTION

Ginseng in the East has been used for centuries as a general medicine and has different effects for different people. Ginseng stimulates the entire body to build resistance against stress, increase energy, and to overcome mental and physical fatigue and weakness. It is beneficial for the heart, circulation and nourishes the brain cells. It is an excellent preventive for diseases and for restoring health after sickness. It improves concentration and has been considered helpful by many people in slowing the aging process. The Chinese have testified for centuries about its beneficial effects on immunity and longevity.

There are two main types of ginseng. Panax is considered to be the genuine ginseng and has two major species, P. ginseng of eastern Asia and P. quinquefolium that grows in North America. Siberian ginseng (Eleutherococcus senticosus) is botanically different from the Panax genus but shares many of the same effects.

Russian scientists tested ginseng on proofreaders who need good concentration powers with high accuracy and speed. Those using ginseng increased their speed by 12 percent and decreased mistakes by an amazing 51 percent in comparison with the readers who did not use ginseng. In Sweden, university students undergoing exams were shown to do better when taking ginseng. In the United States, nurses changing from day to night shifts found that, if taking ginseng, problems of moodiness, insomnia and decreased alertness were relieved.

Some definitive health benefits derived from taking ginseng are improved stamina and concentration, increased resistance to stress, disease, and fatigue, and protection against radiation. Ginseng appears to stimulate the nervous system and thus increase speed and accuracy on various tasks and under different stressors. Tests have shown an increase in learning retention. Ginseng, especially Siberian ginseng, differs from other stimulants, such as caffeine, in that it does not produce the side effects of jitteriness, over-stimulation or subsequent exhaustion.

Ginseng has been shown to reverse and block the effects of alcohol and sedative drugs. It also can have a calming effect and for this reason is commonly used to alleviate stress. A major study over several months involving 60,000 Soviet auto workers showed that use of ginseng produced an improvement in general health. Japanese research scientists found that ginseng seems to strengthen the immune system. Ginseng has even been found to help diabetics.

TOXICITY, CAUTIONS AND CONTRAINDICATIONS

There are no known drug interactions or contraindications for ginseng. Ginseng does not have any reported side effects.

AMERICAN GINSENG
(Panax quinquefolium)

ORIGIN
Canada, and eastern and midwestern US, particularly Wisconsin

PART OF PLANT USED
Root

DESCRIPTION
American ginseng (Panax quinquefolium) is a deciduous perennial shrub, the fleshy root of which requires four years to reach maturity. Traditionally, the wild root was consumed by Native Americans as a general tonic, a natural restorative for the weak and wounded, and to help the mind. American ginseng is now used as a natural preventive and restorative remedy and valued for its adaptogenic properties. American ginseng is more sedative and relaxing and increases "yin" energy while Korean ginseng is more stimulating and increases the "yang" energy. American ginseng is nonetheless suitable for males and females as well as for young and older people.

The main active ingredients of ginseng are the more than 20 saponin triterpenoid glycosides called ginsenosides whose names relate to their chromatographic position (Ra, Rb, etc.). American ginseng is rich in the Rb1 group of ginsenosides which have more sedative and metabolic effects on the central nervous system, compared to the Rg1 group of ginsenosides which are more arousing and stimulating. In addition to its CNS-depressing activity, Rb1 ginsenosides also have weak anti-inflammatory action and increase digestive tract peristalsis. Laboratory animals given Rb1 ginsenosides have improved stamina and increased learning abilities. Other studies have shown that

Rb1 ginsenosides also have antifatigue, anticonvulsant, antipyretic, antipsychotic, analgesic and ulcer protective effects.

American ginseng has been used for stress and fatigue characterized by insomnia, poor appetite, nervousness and restlessness.

TRADITIONAL AND OTHER THERAPEUTIC USES

- CNS depressant, sedative, relaxant, and anti-convulsant, effects
- antistress and hypotensive effects
- antifatigue
- restorative for those with an active, nervous, or agitated disposition
- increases vitality in conditions of weakness, prolonged stress, poor immunity, or chronic disease
- analgesic, anti-inflammatory and antipyretic
- immune system stimulant
- anti-tumor
- regulates blood sugar and lipid levels and adrenal gland function, inhibiting adrenal exhaustion
- increases gastrointestinal mobility
- increases synthesis of cholesterol in liver
- antipsychotic

TOXICITY, CAUTIONS AND CONTRAINDICATIONS

No reported toxicity.

KOREAN GINSENG
(Panax ginseng)

ORIGIN
Asian mountain forests, Korea

PART OF PLANT USED
Root

DESCRIPTION
Panax ginseng is a deciduous perennial shrub whose fleshy root requires four to six years of cultivation to reach maturity. Traditionally, the wild root was consumed to vitalize, strengthen, and rejuvenate the entire body. Widely cultivated, ginseng is now used as a natural preventive, restorative remedy and valued for its adaptogenic properties. Korean ginseng is more stimulating and increases the "yang" energy while American ginseng (Panax quinquefolium) increases the "yin" energy. Korean ginseng is traditionally more suitable for males and older people.

The main active ingredients of ginseng are the more than 20 saponin triterpenoid glycosides called ginsenosides whose names relate to their chromatographic position (Ra, Rb, etc.). The Rb1 group of ginsenosides have more sedative and metabolic effects on the central nervous system, while the Rg1 group of ginsenosides are more arousing and stimulating at low doses. Rb1 ginsenosides have CNS-depressing activity, have weak anti-inflammatory action, and increase digestive tract peristalsis. Other studies have shown that Rb1 ginsenosides also are anticonvulsant, antipyretic, antipsychotic, analgesic, and ulcer protective.

These activities contrast with those of Rg1 ginsenosides, which have weak CNS-stimulating activity, protect against fatigue, and cause an increase in motor activity. Panax ginseng (Korean) contains higher amounts of the more stimulating Rg1 ginsenosides compared to American ginseng (Panax quinquefolium), which has a higher amount of the more sedative Rb1 ginsenosides. Both Rg1 and Rb1 ginsenosides act on the adrenal and pituitary glands and help them respond to stress more rapidly.

TRADITIONAL AND OTHER THERAPEUTIC USES

- adaptogen and general tonic
- antistress and antifatigue restorative and slight CNS stimulant
- increases mental and physical work capacity
- enhances mental acuity and intellectual performance
- improves reaction times
- increases resistance to infections
- regulates adrenal function, helping prevent adrenal exhaustion
- antioxidant
- promotes appetite
- lowers blood cholesterol
- radioprotective

TOXICITY, CAUTIONS AND CONTRAINDICATIONS

No adverse effects have been reported. P. ginseng may cause a mild insomnia if taken at bedtime.

SIBERIAN GINSENG
(Eleutherococcus senticosus)

ORIGIN
China, Russia (eastern Siberia), Manchuria, Korea

PARTS OF PLANT USED
Rhizome (underground creeping stem) and roots

DESCRIPTION
Siberian ginseng is a tall, wild deciduous shrub with many stalks and a woody root, which has been used for 2,000 years in China as a general preventive medicine and tonic. During this century, Siberian ginseng has been extensively studied by Russian scientists. Numerous clinical trials have established that E. senticosus acts as an adaptogen and helps human beings handle stressful conditions and excel in athletic and mental endeavors.

Siberian ginseng is used by deep sea divers, long-distance drivers, mountain rescue workers, factory workers, athletes, submariners and cosmonauts. After nearly a thousand studies, Siberian ginseng has been shown to increase energy and stamina and to help the body resist viral infections, environmental toxins, radiation, and chemotherapy. In Chinese medicine, it has been used to prevent bronchial and other respiratory infections as well as viral infections. It has been used in cardiovascular and neurovascular conditions to help restore memory, concentration, and cognitive abilities, which may be impaired from poor blood supply to the brain.

The eleutherosides, a range of glycosides with aromatic alcohol aglycones, have been shown to be responsible for the adaptogenic properties of the plant. (Ginsenosides have triterpenoid aglycones.) The glycosides appear to act on the adrenal glands, helping to prevent adrenal hypertrophy and excess corticosteroid production in response to stress.

TRADITIONAL AND OTHER THERAPEUTIC USES

- adaptogen
- reduces stress, fights fatigue, and restores vigor
- treats neurasthenia, debility, depression, and nervous exhaustion
- increases mental and physical work capacity
- stimulates and regulates the immune system, thus helping resist infections
- normalizes hypo- and hyperglycemia
- relieve allergies, hayfever
- reduce convalescence time
- protect against environmental toxins and pollution
- promote appetite
- increase fertility

TOXICITY, CAUTIONS AND CONTRAINDICATIONS

No toxicity or side effects have been reported. It should not be taken with a high fever (above 39° C or 102° F) or at a very high blood pressure (WHO stage 2).

GOLDENSEAL
(Hydrastis canadensis)

ORIGIN
Northern America

PART OF PLANT USED
Rhizome (root-stock)

DESCRIPTION
Goldenseal root (Hydrastis canadensis) has been used by Native American healers for a wide range of ailments. They used goldenseal for local inflammations and infections. The plant was also utilized to improve digestion as a bitter tonic and to treat ulcers. An infusion of the root was used as a soothing rinse for eye and skin infections.

Goldenseal root has been recommended for a variety of inflamed mucous membranes, including stomach, intestinal, vaginal, and rectal. It has been reported that the plant relieves pain and helps heal wounds and stop bleeding. In addition, the antibacterial action helps reduce or prevent infection of open sores. Native Americans of the Cherokee and Iroquois tribes used the plant for diarrhea, dyspepsia, liver problems, flatulence, pneumonia, cancer, and rattlesnake bites. In modern times it has been used as a laxative and diuretic, and as a treatment for hemorrhoids, mouth sores, infections, acne, and sore throats.

The active ingredients of goldenseal include a group of alkaloids, hydrastine and berberine. These alkaloids are strongly astringent and help reduce inflammation of mucous membranes.

TRADITIONAL AND OTHER THERAPEUTIC USES
- treats inflammation of digestive system and mucous membranes

- treats peptic ulcers, gastritis, flatulence, diarrhea, dyspepsia
- for liver and gall bladder problems
- douche for candidiasis and thrush
- treats skin infections, impetigo, ringworm, eczema
- lowers blood pressure
- promotes rest and sleep
- treats vaginitis, gonorrhea, urethritis and rectal inflammations
- treats rhinitis and catarrhal conditions of the common cold and flu
- treats eye inflammations
- treast disturbances of endocrine function
- treats excessive menstruation and uterine hemorrhaging

TOXICITY, CAUTIONS AND CONTRAINDICATIONS

At doses of two to three grams, goldenseal can lower heart rate, and at higher doses it can be paralyzing to the central nervous system (CNS). Do not use during pregnancy since berberine stimulates the uterus and may induce abortion at high doses.

GOTU KOLA
(Centella asiatica l.)

ORIGIN
Madagascar (wild)

PART OF PLANT USED
Aerial portion

DESCRIPTION
Centella is actually a specific variety of gotu kola, but since no other varieties possess such high amounts of asiaticosides and other triterpenes, the term "centella" is reserved for just this variety and "gotu kola" is used for all other varieties. Centella is found only in Madagascar while the other varieties of gotu kola are found in India and neighboring countries. Centella does not contain caffeine or any derivatives.

Asiaticosides stimulate the reticuloendothelial system where new blood cells are formed and old ones destroyed, fatty materials are stored, iron is metabolized and immune responses and inflammation begin. The primary mode of action of Centella appears to be on the various phases of connective tissue development, which are part of the healing process. Centella also increases keratinization, the process of building more skin in areas of infection such as sores and ulcers. Asiaticosides also stimulate the synthesis of lipids and proteins necessary for healthy skin. Finally, Centella strengthens veins by repairing the connective tissues surrounding veins and decreasing capillary fragility.

Centella has been found to have important healing effects on solid tissues, including skin, connective tissues, lymph tissues, blood vessels, and mucous membranes. It has found its most successful applications in the treatment of conditions involving venous insufficiency, tissue inflammation and infection, and post-surgical healing. Preparations can be applied topically or taken internally.

TRADITIONAL AND OTHER THERAPEUTIC USES

- treats skin injuries such as open wounds, sores, tears, cuts, and ulcers,
- alleviates bed sores, thrombophlebitis, tingling, nocturnal cramps and other results of confinement
- phlebitis, varicose veins, cellulite, edema and other conditions of venous insufficiency
- various skin infections such as cellulites, erysipelas, and radiation ulcers
- useful for perineal lesions and episiotomy tears occurring during delivery and obstetric manipulation and other gynecological problems
- sedative tonic which is said to improve learning and memory

GRAPE SEED EXTRACT
(Vitis vinifera)

ORIGIN
Europe

PART OF PLANT USED
Seed

DESCRIPTION
Grape seed extract is an antioxidant-rich extract, especially high in bioflavonoids, which is used for fighting free radicals and maintaining capillary health. It is very similar to pine bark extract, with a high content of proanthocyanidins. These are found in many foods, but freezing, cooking and canning deactivate them.

Grape seed extract is used for its free radical-fighting capabilities, and for a variety of conditions related to capillary health and permeability. It is synergistic with vitamin C, which is more potent and absorbed more rapidly when used together with proanthocyanidins.

Free radicals do damage in the capillaries in two ways. They inactivate a compound called a 1-antitripsin, whose role is to restrain the enzymes that break down collagen, elastin and hyaluronic acid. They also turn fats in the cell membranes rancid by lipid peroxidation. Proanthocyanidins protect both the 1-antitripsin and the lipids by neutralizing the specific types of free radicals most likely to damage them, and may also directly inhibit the damaging enzymes. Collagen, elastin and hyaluronic acid make up much of the inner wall and supporting matrix of the capillaries. When they are in good shape the capillaries stretch to let red blood cells through the tight places and do not let the fluids in the blood leak out.

Proanthocyanidins (also known as leucoan-thocyanidins) are a form of polyphenol, which is in turn a form of bioflavonoid. Proanthocyanidins are at least 15 to 25 times more powerful than vitamin E in neutralizing the iron and oxygen species free radicals that attack lipids.

TRADITIONAL AND OTHER THERAPEUTIC USES

- poor distribution of microcirculatory blood flow in the brain and heart
- altered capillary fragility and permeability, especially in diabetes mellitus
- chronic arterial/venous insufficiency in the extremities
- altered platelet aggregation and other charac-teristics of blood flow in capillaries
- breakdown in the elastic fibers of the capillaries (collagen and elastin) due to free radical and enzyme action
- microangiopathy of the retina, edema of the lymph nodes, and varicose veins
- cumulative effects of aging, reducing the risk of degenerative diseases

TOXICITY, CAUTIONS AND CONTRAINDICATIONS

Proanthocyanidins are almost completely non-toxic both in acute dosage and long-term use. They have no known potential for causing mutation or birth defects, and have no adverse effect on fertility, pregnancy or nursing.

GREEN TEA
(Camellia sinensis)

ORIGIN
Asia

PART OF PLANT USED
Leaf

DESCRIPTION
Green tea is composed of natural dried leaves of the tea plant, Camellia sinensis. Black tea is oxidized green tea. Both have been used for thousands of years in Asia as a beverage and as medicine. Green tea extract is bioflavonoid-rich and potent, used primarily for fighting free radicals. It has a high content of polyphenols, which are a class of bioflavonoids.

The polyphenols in green tea are catechins, with multiple linked ring-like structures. Polyphenols are a form of bioflavonoids with several phenol groups. They determine both taste and biological action of the specific tea. The dominant and most important catechin in green tea is epigallocatechin gallate (EGCG), a potent antioxidant, which is used for food production as well as in animal research studies. The phenol groups capture pro-oxidants and free radicals. EGCG is over 200 times more powerful than vitamin E in neutralizing the pro-oxidants and free radicals that attack lipids in the brain, in vivo. It is 20 times more potent than vitamin E in reducing formation of peroxides in lard by the Active Oxygen Method, in vitro.

Though green tea extract is used primarily for its free radical-fighting capabilities, it has a wide range of applications. Its key ingredient, EGCG, protects against digestive and respiratory infections. In one study, a solution of 1 mcg per ml of EGCG in vitro significantly inhibited influenza virus. It helps block the cancer-promoting actions of carcinogens, ultraviolet light, and metastasis from an original site in the skin, stomach, small intestine, liver or lung. Higher quantities (0.5 percent to 1 percent of the diet) were protective against high total and LDL-cholesterol in rats placed on cholesterol-promoting diets. Crude catechins at 0.5 percent of the diet were effective in lowering blood pressures in spontaneously hypertensive rats. Both EGCG and black tea catechins suppressed angiotensin I converting enzyme, which causes essential hypertension. EGCG also reduces platelet aggregation about as much as aspirin or Ginkgo biloba extract. Green tea is very effective in inhibiting pathogenic bacteria that cause food poisoning, but increases levels of acidophilus (friendly) bacteria. 500 mg of catechin (i.e. 250 mg EGCG) daily significantly helps make bowel habits regular. Green tea also blocks the attachment of bacteria associated with dental caries to the teeth.

TRADITIONAL AND OTHER THERAPEUTIC USES

- primarily used for its free radical-fighting capabilities
- helps block the cancer-promoting actions of chemical carcinogens, ultraviolet light, and metastasis
- high total and LDL-cholesterol levels
- high blood pressure (suppresses angiotensin I converting enzyme)
- reduces platelet aggregation
- inhibits pathogenic bacteria that cause food poisoning
- blocks the attachment of the bacteria associated with dental caries to the teeth
- supplies the mineral, manganese

TOXICITY, CAUTIONS AND CONTRAINDICATIONS

Green tea extract is non-toxic both in acute dosage and in long-term use (no significant effect on weight gain at two percent of the diet in three months in rats). It has no potential for causing mutations or birth defects, and has no adverse effect on fertility, pregnancy or nursing.

GUARANA
(Paullinia cupana)

ORIGIN
South America, especially Brazilian rain forests

PART OF PLANT USED
Seeds

DESCRIPTION
Guarana is a caffeine-rich beverage from South America. Sometimes known as "Brazilian cocoa," guarana is made into a popular cola drink, which is drunk in Brazil for energy and stimulation. Guarana is a creeping shrub whose seeds have been used medicinally for centuries by the native inhabitants as an energizer, stimulant and intestinal cleanser.

Guarana has tonifying and astringent properties, particularly on the intestines. It is a natural stimulant due to its content of xanthines. These xanthines include mainly guaranine (natural caffeine), theobromine, and theophylline. Guarana contains two to three times more caffeine than coffee or tea. The caffeine and xanthines have a stimulating effect on the central nervous and circulatory systems.

Guarana has been used as a stimulant, diuretic, and antidiarrheal agent. Other applications have included use as a nervine tonic, anti-fatigue stimulant, to reduce hunger, to relieve headaches including migraines, to alleviate PMS symptoms, and as an aphrodisiac.

TRADITIONAL AND OTHER THERAPEUTIC USES
- fights fatigue
- used as a nervine tonic
- useful against diarrhea and other gastrointestinal

complaints
- alleviates PMS symptoms and listlessness
- quells hunger
- aphrodisiac
- used as a systemic cleanser
- useful in treating neuralgia and other mild pains and headaches

TOXICITY, CAUTIONS AND CONTRAINDICATIONS

Guarana is a caffeine-rich substance, therefore do not overuse and avoid during pregnancy. Dysuria is a common side effect of guarana use.

GUGUL
(Commiphora mukul)

ORIGIN
India

PART OF PLANT USED
Gum resin

DESCRIPTION
Gugul, particularly resin from the Commiphora mukul tree, is widely used in traditional Indian Ayurvedic medicine. After 2,500 years of successful use, this herb from north-central India is making its way into the arsenal of alternative practitioners. The high-quality standardized gugul extracts of today make it a viable alternative in the treatment of cholesterol abnormalities and obesity.

The active component of gugul is the sterols E- and Z-gugulsterone. These compounds have been studied for a variety of metabolic effects, but gugulsterones have been noted for their anti-inflammatory effect. Glucosamine sulfate is recognized in Europe as a chondroprotective agent, which is a substance that increases chondrocyte anabolic activity (International Journal of Tissue Reactions, vol. 14(5) pg. 231, 1992). Although people report excellent results in the long run from glucosamines, they exert no anti-inflammatory activity. Because of this, gugul is a viable complement to glucosamine sulfate for treating arthritis.

A study in Drugs of Today found 79 percent of 245 patients who had high cholesterol experienced a 27 percent drop in cholesterol and a 22 percent drop in triglycerides using Gugul. While many people need to reduce dietary intake of fats to control obesity, this can result in a lowering of HDL ("good" cholesterol) as well as LDL and Very Low Density Lipoproteins. Also, less lipid-soluble vitamins such as beta carotene, retinol (vitamin A), toco-pherol (vitamin E), and vitamins D and K might be less well absorbed. The Indian Journal of Medicine reported results of a 16-week trial analyzing the effects of gugul on HDL. In summary, HDL levels increased by 35 percent!

TRADITIONAL AND OTHER THERAPEUTIC USES
- lowers LDL cholesterol while raising HDL cholesterol
- controls and reduce obesity
- complements glucosamine sulfate and boswella in treating inflammation of arthritis

TOXICITY, CAUTIONS AND CONTRAINDICATIONS

In the north Indian state of Jammu, the Regional Research Laboratories investigated gugul for its effect on rheumatic diseases and found it to be free of any "adverse and undesirable side-effects." The high-quality standardized gugul extracts of today make it a viable adjunct in the treatment of cholesterol abnormalities and obesity. Before making any changes, however, it is wise to confer with a physician.

GYMNEMA
(Gymnema sylvestre)

ORIGIN

India

PARTS OF PLANT USED

Leaves and roots

DESCRIPTION

Gymnema sylvestre is a woody, vine-like plant which climbs on bushes and trees in the Western Ghats in South India, and to the west of those mountains in the territory around the coastal city of Goa. It came to be known as "destroyer of sugar" because, in ancient times, Ayurvedic physicians observed that chewing a few leaves of Gymnema suppressed the taste of sugar. That is, sweet foods no longer tasted sweet, but rather became almost completely tasteless. In later generations, clinical tests showed that regular use over a period of three to four months helped to reduce glycosuria, or the appearance of sugar in the urine. Recent clinical trials conducted in India have shown that an extract of G. sylvestre is useful in both insulin-dependent diabetes mellitus (IDDM) and in certain types of non-insulin-dependent diabetes mellitus (NIDDM). As a result of these clinical tests and years of successful treatments, Gymnema is used today all over India for treating diabetes mellitus. In reducing the symptom of glycosuria, the dried leaves are used in daily doses of three to four grams for a period of three months or more.

Studies conducted in India as early as 1930 showed that the leaves of G. sylvestre cause hypoglycemia in experimental animals. This state of hypoglycemia is explained on the assumption that the drug indirectly stimulates insulin secretion of the pancreas, since it has no direct effect on carbohydrate metabolism.

Recent pharmacological and clinical studies have shown that Gymnema sylvestre acts on two sites, the taste buds in the oral cavity50 and the absorptive surface to the intestines. The structure of the taste buds, which detect sugar in the mouth, is similar to the structure of the tissue that absorbs sugar in the intestine. The important active ingredient of G. sylvestre is an organic acid called "gymnemic acid." The gymnemic acid is made up of molecules whose arrangement is similar to that of glucose molecules. Those molecules fill the receptor locations on the taste buds for a period of one to two hours, thereby preventing the taste buds from being activated by any sugar molecules present in the food. Similarly, the glucose-like molecules in the gymnemic acid fill the receptor locations in the absorptive external layers of the intestine, thereby preventing the intestine from absorbing the sugar molecules.

It has also been noted that Gymnema sylvestre takes away the bitter taste of bitter substances, such as quinine, in much the same way that it affects the sense of sweetness associated with candies and other sweet foods. However, it has no effect on pungent, salty, astringent or acidic tastes. Therefore, if you are eating an orange within two hours after chewing Gymnema sylvestre leaves, for instance, you would taste the sourness of it but not the sweetness.

TRADITIONAL AND OTHER THERAPEUTIC USES

- suppress the taste of sweet foods, and consequently the desire to eat
- reduce metabolic effects of sugar by preventing the intestines from absorbing sugar molecules during digestion
- treatment of diabetes
- snakebite treated by powder or paste of the root applied to the wound

- fever treated with oral administration of half an ounce to an ounce (one part in 10) of leaves
- swollen glands treated with an external application of triturated leaves mixed with castor oil

TOXICITY, CAUTIONS AND CONTRAINDICATIONS

For most people using G. sylvestre, blood sugar goes down toward but not below normal blood sugar levels. This can happen in a small number of patients, however, because the mechanisms of the diabetic syndrome vary with different patients. Remarkably, unlike insulin or oral hypoglycemic sulfonylurea compounds, the hypoglycemic effects of Gymnema sylvestre are seen in only a small percentage of diabetic patients. The safety of Gymnema sylvestre has been demonstrated by the fact that it has been safely and successfully used for more than 2,000 years in traditional Ayurvedic medicine.

HORNY GOAT WEED

DESCRIPTION

The Chinese consider horny goat weed as the premier herb to increase libido in both men and women, and an excellent enhancer of erectile function in men. The plant has long been employed to restore sexual "fire", boost erectile function, allay fatigue and even alleviate menopausal discomfort. Horny goat weed was first described in classic Chinese medicinal texts dating back more than 2,000 years as a sexual enhancer. The Chinese use the term Yin Yang Huo in reference to any of several species of epimedium, a leafy groundcover that grows most abundantly at high altitude. The leaves contain a variety of flavonoids, polysaccharides, lignans, and other substances.

Horny goat weed got its name hundreds of years ago, when a goat herder noticed his male goats were especially raucous, mounting their mates several times during a brief period. Curious, the young man observed the animals carefully. He noticed that whenever they ate from a certain patch of weeds, their promiscuous behavior became more pronounced several hours afterwards.

This remarkable herb seems custom-made by nature for the flagging male and female libido, especially when combined with certain other herbs. Additionally, Yin Yang Huo has been shown to stimulate the adrenal glands, triggering increased hormonal secretions. Research has shown that male sperm count and semen density increase substantially with its use.

Yin Yang Huo may also expand the circulatory system's blood vessels, while allowing hormone-enriched blood to penetrate sensitive tissues. The Chinese claim this improved circulation eliminates tiredness and increases energy, while nervous stimulation is boosted as the brain is flooded with hormone-rich blood.

TRADITIONAL AND OTHER THERAPEUTIC USES

A powerful sexual enhancer for both men and women

TOXICITY. CAUTIONS AND CONTRAINDICATIONS

No known toxicity.

HAWTHORN
(Crategus oxyancantha)

ORIGIN
Britain, Europe, North America

PART OF PLANT USED
Berries

DESCRIPTION
Hawthorn is a small thorny tree with white or red flowers and berries. It is one of the most valuable cardiovascular tonics available. The berries are rich in flavonoids, which have been shown to dilate peripheral and coronary blood vessels. This action helps alleviate hypertension and high blood pressure and reduce the severity and frequency of angina attacks. Hawthorn also is a rich source of procyanidins, which have sedative and antispasmodic effects.

TRADITIONAL AND OTHER THERAPEUTIC USES
- acts as a cardiotonic, restoring both high and low blood pressure to normal
- treats irregular heartbeats and arterial spasms (Raynaud's)
- used in certain nervous disorders, such as insomnia

TOXICITY, CAUTIONS AND CONTRAINDICATIONS
There is no known toxicity, but hawthorn may potentiate the action of digitalis.

WITCH HAZEL
(Hamamelis virginiana)

ORIGIN
North America, Atlantic region

PARTS OF PLANT USED
Bark and twigs

DESCRIPTION
Hemorrhoids are among the worst gastrointestinal problems and one of the most common digestive disorders in the industrialized world. It seems that the combination of poor diet, lack of exercise, and stress-filled lifestyles leads to this particular brand of nightmare. The good news is that hemorrhoids are readily treated with herbal medicine.

'Heme' refers to blood, and hemorrhoids are a disorder of the vessels that carry the blood, specifically, "a vascular tumor made up of infected varices of the veins of the hemorrhoidal plexus." They are called external or internal hemorrhoids, external piles being within the sphincter ani. An external hemorrhoid consists of an extravasation of blood from a ruptured vein, which forms a hard mass in the surrounding cellular tissues. Internal hemorrhoids are caused by a dilation of the hemorrhoidal arteries and veins, which become varicose and form tumors. More simply put, a hemorrhoid is a blood vessel that has ballooned up and out of shape. Rather than operating as a pipe for blood to run through, the blood vessel becomes a pool. As blood fills this pool, the vessel hardens into a little ball. The swollen blood vessels press on nerve endings, which send messages to the brain, resulting in unpleasant sensations.

Like all of our other digestive problems, hemorrhoids are linked to stress. In fact, stress scientists believe that hemorrhoids are a stress-related illness. The theory is that when people are stressed out, they clench their muscles, including those in the anal area.

Witch hazel is a rather peculiar tree, which breaks into bloom in the dead of winter, producing threadlike strings of bright yellow petals that simply hang off the bark at irregular intervals. The Native Americans were familiar with this woodland tree, which can be found growing from New Brunswick to Florida, and they were in the habit of using it to reduce inflammations of all sorts, especially with wounds. The life of the Native Americans was an extremely physical one, and whether the injury came from a battle wound or from a slide down a mountaintop, they found that a poultice of witch hazel would ease the pain and speed the healing process.

TRADITIONAL AND OTHER THERAPEUTIC USES

- treats wounds and external inflammations, including hemorrhoids

HOPS
(Humulus lupulus)

ORIGIN
Netherlands, North American, Europe

PART OF PLANT USED
Female strobiles (fruit)

DESCRIPTION
The hops plant is a hedgerow climber with a tendency to twine around trees. The plant has been used since Roman times in brewing and as a traditional nervine and sedative herb. Hops tea has been recommended for insomnia, restlessness, and diarrhea. In addition, a hops pillow was frequently used in the past for the sedative effects of the volatile oils released while sleeping.

Extensive modern research indicates that hops can relax smooth muscle tissue as well as act as a sedative. The bitter acids, lupulone and humulone, are some of the identified active ingredients with sedative properties. The flavonglucosides have diuretic and spasmolytic properties. In addition, estrogenic substances have been identified in hops and it is an anaphrodisiac.

Hops have been used to treat digestive tract disorders involving spasms of the smooth muscle, especially irritable bowel syndrome and Crohn's disease.

TRADITIONAL AND OTHER THERAPEUTIC USES
- treats insomnia, nervous tension, and restlessness
- aids in cases of hysteria
- used to treat intestinal spasms, Crohn's disease, and irritable bowel syndrome
- anti-inflammatory
- anaphrodisiac

- stimulates appetite
- aids in treating climacteric disorders (e.g. menopause)
- mild diuretic
- increases breast milk for irritable infants

TOXICITY, CAUTIONS AND CONTRAINDICATIONS

There is no known toxicity. Large quantities can have an anaphrodisiac effect. Female hops pickers have suffered from loss of menstruation as a result of absorbing the oil through their hands. Hops are not recommended for persons suffering from depressive illness.

HORSETAIL
(Equisetum arvense)

ORIGIN
Europe

PART OF PLANT USED
Herb (above ground portion)

DESCRIPTION
Horsetail grass is a plant made up of bunches of leafless tubular stems or rushes. The plant grows in moist soil and concentrates minerals, particularly silica. The plant is also valued for its astringent and antibiotic properties. In folklore practices, horsetail grass was used to accelerate the healing of broken bones and connective tissue injuries and to promote healthy eyes, hair, skin and nails.

The essential element, silicon, is present in very large amounts in horsetail grass. The element is present in the plant in its organic forms, silicon dioxide ($SiO2$) or silicic acid/silicate ($Si(OH)2$). Silica is essential for growth and healing, being a major constituent of bones, cartilage, connective tissue and skin. In the body silica makes up part of the mucopolysaccharides (glycosaminoglycans), which play critical structural roles in bone and cartilage. The degeneration of tissues with age corresponds with decreasing levels of silica in the tissue. Silicic acid also stimulates an increase in white blood cells, helping to increase resistance to infection. In the past a tea of horsetail grass was frequently given to tuberculosis patients. The second major class of ingredients of horsetail grass is the saponins. These compounds have a mild diuretic effect. Horsetail is widely used for genitourinary problems including inflammations, kidney or other stones, enuresis, nephritis, gout and prostate problems.

TRADITIONAL AND OTHER THERAPEUTIC USES

- mild diuretic
- improves broken nails, lifeless hair, hair loss, and skin disorders
- treats anemia
- useful for general debility
- helps to stop bleeding
- useful for stomach ulcers
- shrinks inflamed or enlarged prostate
- cystitis and urinary stones
- lung complaints
- arteriosclerosis
- pulmonary tuberculosis
- strengthens the immune system
- used as an ingredient in shampoos and cosmetics

TOXICITY, CAUTIONS AND CONTRAINDICATIONS

Horsetail has no known toxic effect with normal use. Avoid its use with antihypertensive drugs, digitalis, corticosteroids, heparin or lithium.

KAVA KAVA
(Piper methysticum)

ORIGIN
South Pacific

PART OF PLANT USED
Root

DESCRIPTION
Kava kava root has been used in the South Pacific cultures for centuries as a relaxant herb, and is still widely used. In this ethnobotanical context, the resinous juice is extracted from the root and made into a beverage. The explorer, Captain James Cook, gave Kava its botanical name, which means, "intoxicating pepper." To make standardized extracts for use in Europe and the United States, cultivated kava has been selectively reproduced over many generations from wild root stocks of plants that contain high levels of activity.

Research into the source of kava's activity has been ongoing for over 100 years. It is now widely accepted that the active compounds are a group of 15 lactones unique to the plant, and referred to as kavalactones. There are also some alkaloids present, but it is not known whether or not these are responsible for any of kava's activity. Bio-enhancing agents include valerian root, hops, chamomile, and licorice.

TRADITIONAL AND OTHER THERAPEUTIC USES
- relaxant and sleep aid
- mildly psychoactive properties, which induce feelings of peace, contentment, and sharpened senses

TOXICITY, CAUTIONS AND CONTRAINDICATIONS
There are none known.

KOLA NUT (COLA)
{Cola acuminata (P. beauv.)
Cola nitida}

ORIGIN
Tropical Africa

PART OF PLANT USED
Seed kernel

DESCRIPTION
Cola (also kola and cola nut) is the seed kernel of a large African tree, Cola acuminata (P. beauv.) or Cola nitida (Schott. & Endl), of the Sterculiaceae family, commercially grown around the world in the tropics as a caffeine stimulant. The nuts are basically round, 1/4- to 3/4-inch long, flattened and rounded on one side, irregularly scooped out on the other side, occurring in pairs. They start out white and turn a characteristic red or reddish gray when dried.

Cola stimulates the central nervous system, and as such is an antidepressant. It also has astringent and diuretic properties. It may relieve some migraine headaches. It may have antioxidant activities due to its phenolic and anthrocyanin constituents.

Key constituents are caffeine, with traces of theobromine; tannins and phenolics, including d-catechin, 1-epicatechin, kolatin, and kolanin (catechol and (-) epicatechol are lost on drying); phlobaphene and anthocyanin pigment, kola red; betaine; protein; and starch.

TRADITIONAL AND OTHER THERAPEUTIC USES
- augments the capacity for physical exertion
- increases power, especially in enduring fatigue without food

- counteracts nervous debility, states of atony and weakness, nervous diarrhea, depression, anorexia, and sea sickness
- gives rise to euphoric states in some people
- useful in treating some varieties of migraine headache, but is unlikely to bring relief to those who regularly drink coffee or other caffeinated drinks
- may give a lift to those suffering from neurasthenia and hysteria, characterized by great mental despondency, foreboding, and brooding
- especially indicated if the heart is feeble and irregular in its action, with general muscular feebleness

TOXICITY, CAUTIONS AND CONTRAINDICATIONS

Kola nut is not considered toxic. A 1901 text says, "Not infrequently, however, connected thought is rendered more difficult" as impressions become too fleeting. Do not use when caffeine is contraindicated.

LICORICE
(Glycyrrhiza glabra, G. uralensis)

ORIGIN
Europe, Asia

PART OF PLANT USED
Root

DESCRIPTION
The leguminous plant, Glycyrrhiza glabra, contains a substance, glycyrrhizin, which is 50 times sweeter than sugar. Sugar, as we know it today, is a relatively new development; 400 years ago, the only sweet tastes came from fruit and honey. The extreme sweetness of licorice made it a real oddity, and people loved it. Due to its peculiar sweetness, licorice was used in many medicines to mask the unpleasant taste of the other ingredients. This is still a common practice in China today.

There are two kinds of licorice used in herbal medicinals, G. glabra, which is the European variety, and G. uralensis, which is the Chinese variety. Licorice has been used for centuries. Apparently the Greeks first obtained the sweet roots from the Scythians. Theophrastus, a Greek writer in the third century B.C., noted the Scythian root's value in treating asthma, dry coughs, and anything else troubling the respiratory system. King Tut's tomb was said to be loaded with licorice.

Dioscorides, another ancient writer on herbal medicine, called the plant glycyrrhiza. This means "sweet root," which indeed licorice is. The Romans called the plant liquiritia, which became the English word, 'licorice.' The Roman writers Celsus, Scribonius, and Largus all mention the plant. Like the Greeks, they found the root to be amazingly effective in quieting an irritating cough.

Roman soldiers are said to have carried licorice with them on their moves northward to countries where coughs and colds due to harsh weather were so common. Licorice was used in Germany during the Middle Ages. The English King Henry IV kept a good supply in his pharmacy, as records dating to 1424 indicate. An Italian medical writer named Saladinus states that licorice could be found in all the pharmacies of 15th-century Italy. Though other European countries grew the plant, the Italian root was said to be the best for both medicine and candy. As a cough treatment, licorice has been in active use for at least 2,300 years.

Licorice is one of the most popular medicinal herbs in China. The Chinese consider it to be antitussive, demulcent, emollient, expectorant, and a mild laxative. It is used to treat coughs, consumption, laryngitis, sore throat, bronchitis, and chronic bronchitis.

The Chinese have found at least ten anti-inflammatory flavonoids in licorice, along with an acid, glycyrrhetic acid, that has been proven to be both antibacterial and antitussive. This triple combination makes licorice perfect for the job at hand. In fact, licorice's anti-inflammatory abilities are so strong that they are used to heal all manner of irritated tissues be they inside or on the surface of the body. The action is very much like that of a steroid such as cortisone. The good news with this steroid-like action is that it does not come with the immune-suppressing side effects of chemically synthesized steroids. People who are attempting to taper off corticosteroids often use licorice to help wean their bodies.

TRADITIONAL AND OTHER THERAPEUTIC USES
- cough suppression and bronchial soothing
- heals internal and external irritated tissues

TOXICITY, CAUTIONS AND CONTRAINDICATIONS

The U.S. Food and Drug Administration has rated licorice "generally recognized as safe."

MACA
(Peruvian Ginseng, Maka)

DESCRIPTION

Maca is a hardy perennial plant cultivated high in the Andean Mountains. It has one of the highest frost tolerances among native cultivated species. Maca is propagated by seed. Although it is a perennial, it is grown as an annual, and 7-9 months from planting are required to produce the harvested roots.

Maca has been used medicinally for centuries to enhance fertility in humans and animals. This energizing plant is also referred to as Peruvian ginseng.

Maca has a large amount of essential amino acids and higher levels of iron and calcium than potatoes. It contains important amounts of fatty acids including linolenic, palmitic, and oleic acids. Research on maca indicates that the effects on fertility are a result of the glucosinolates.

Maca is growing in world popularity due to its energizing effects, fertility enhancement and aphrodisiac qualities. Other traditional uses include increasing energy, stamina and endurance in athletes, promoting mental clarity, treating male impotence and helping with menstural irregularities. It is also a good tonic for menopause and chronic fatigue syndrome.

It is used as an alternative to anabolic steroids by bodybuilders due to its richness in sterols. It acts on men to restore them to a healthy functional status in which they experience a more active libido by normalizing testosterone, progesterone and estrogen levels. Maca has a lot of easily absorbable calcium, magnesium and a fair amount of silica.

TRADITIONAL AND OTHER THERAPEUTIC USES

- male impotence
- erectile dysfunction
- menopausal symptoms
- general fatigue; increases stamina and athletic performance

TOXICITY, CAUTIONS AND CONTRAINDICATIONS

Not known.

MARSHMALLOW
(Althaea officinalis)

ORIGIN
Europe, Asia Minor, and western and northern Asia

PARTS OF PLANT USED
Leaves and root

DESCRIPTION
The marshmallow belongs to a very 'slimy' group of plants, the mallow family, which includes okra, cotton, hibiscus and hollyhock. The common denominator with these plants is their production of a viscous slime. If you have ever eaten okra, or bindi as it is called in Indian cuisine, you are familiar with the substance in question. One thousand species of mallows have been discovered around the globe and all have this slimy quality to a greater or lesser degree.

The mucilage in mallow plants is a complex sugar composed of a number of polysaccharides. One of these is made up of 1-rhamnose, d-galactose, d-galactrunoic acid and d-glucuronic acid. The structure of the polysaccharides contained in marshmallow is such that they cannot be digested by the human body. Beyond polysaccharides, the root contains pectin, asparagines, and tannins.

Marshmallow is the most famous of the mallow family for soothing irritated tissues. The indigestible nature of its mucilage means that when you are taking marshmallow for internal irritations, the slime will slither its way down the entire digestive tract, soothing as it goes and guaranteeing relief from top to bottom.

The leaves of the marshmallow plant as well as the root are used as medicine. Marshmallow leaves are of a slightly different chemical makeup. They contain the same

mucilage as the roots, but they also come packing flavonoids including kaempferol, quercetin and diosmetin
glucosides. Additionally, the leaves contain the coumarin
scopoletin and phenolic acids including syringic acid, caffeic acid and vanillic acid.

TRADITIONAL AND OTHER THERAPEUTIC USES

- internal uses of marshmallow include healing
  irritated respiratory, digestive and urinary
  systems, where it acts as a soothing anti-
  inflammatory
- externally applied, it treats abscesses, boils,
  varicose veins, ulcers, inflammations of the mouth
  and throat, inflamed hemorrhoids, wounds, burns,
  scalds, and bedsores
- paste of marshmallow and slippery elm is applied
  to a splinter, thorn, or even a bee stinger, drawing
  it out and taking away the pain, inflammation, and
  swelling
- poultice treats a variety of wounds

TOXICITY, CAUTIONS AND CONTRAINDICATIONS

Marshmallow was described by Dioscorides 2,000
years ago, so we are fairly safe in saying that it has been
used as an herbal medicinal from the earliest periods.

MILK THISTLE
(Silybum marianum L. gaertn. or Carduus marianus L)

ORIGIN
North America, Europe, moderate climates

PART OF PLANT USED
Seeds

DESCRIPTION
Milk thistle was named Silybum by Dioscorides in 100 A.D. for its large purple, thistle-like flower heads. Since ancient times, the plant was valued for its nutritional and medicinal properties. By the Middle Ages the seed of the milk thistle was commonly used to treat liver diseases, to promote the flow of bile, and as a general tonic for the stomach, spleen, gall bladder, female organs, and liver.

Milk thistle contains three potent liver protective flavonoids, silybin, silydianin and silychristin, known collectively as silymarin. Numerous clinical trials have shown that silymarin and milk thistle extract can protect the liver. Silymarin counteracts the toxic effects of a wide variety of poisons, including alcohol, carbon tetrachloride, acetaminophen overdose, and the deathcap mushroom, Amanito (or Amanita) phalloides which causes death within a day. The mechanism of action of silymarin involves altering the membranes of hepatic cells to inhibit passage of toxins and increasing cellular regeneration by stimulating protein synthesis. Silymarin also has antioxidant activity and inhibits inflammatory enzymes. Recent research has indicated that silymarin helps to protect against depletion of the antioxidant glutathione in liver cells.

Milk thistle extract has been the subject of numerous clinical trials and studies due to its potent liver protective properties. Milk thistle has been used for viral and other forms of hepatitis, cirrhosis, jaundice, and fatty degeneration of the liver. Milk thistle has been used for indigestion since it promotes the flow of bile and thus helps emulsify fats. A positive therapeutic effect has been reported using silymarin for psoriasis. The Eclectics recommended milk thistle for varicose veins.

TRADITIONAL AND OTHER THERAPEUTIC USES
- treats liver disease and acute and chronic hepatitis
- protects the liver from toxins, heavy metals, alcohol, and poisons
- cholagogue
- treats jaundice
- treats psoriasis
- as a uterine tonic, aids in menstrual difficulties
- tonic for the spleen, kidney, and gall bladder
- treats varicose veins

TOXICITY, CAUTIONS AND CONTRAINDICATIONS
No known toxicity, even in large doses.

MUIRA PUAMA
(PTYCHOPETALUM OLACOIDES)

DESCRIPTION

One of the best herbs to use for treating erectile dysfunction or lack of libido is Muira puama (Ptychopetalum olacoides), which is also known as "potency wood." This shrub is native to Brazil and has long been used as a powerful aphrodisiac and nerve-stimulant in South American folk medicine. A recent clinical study has validated its safety and effectiveness in improving libido and sexual function in some patients.

In 1990, a clinical study was conducted at the Institute of Sexology in Paris, France, under the supervision of one of the world's foremost authorities on sexual function, Dr. Jacques Waynberg. Of the 262 subjects who initially complained of lack of sexual desire and the inability to attain or maintain an erection, many of them found Muira puama extract (6:1) to be effective. Within two weeks, at a daily dose of 1 to 1.5 grams of the extract, sixty-two percent of patients with loss of libido claimed that the treatment had a dynamic effect, while fifty-one percent of patients with "erection failures" felt that Muira puama was of benefit.

It appears that Muira puama works on enhancing both psychological and physical aspects of sexual function. Future research will undoubtedly shed additional light on this extremely promising herb.

TRADITIONAL AND OTHER THERAPEUTIC USES
- impotency
- sexual function

TOXICITY, CAUTIONS AND CONTRAINDICATIONS

None noted.

NETTLES
(Urtica dioica)

ORIGIN
Europe, Israel

PART OF PLANT USED
Leaves of young plants

DESCRIPTION
Stinging nettles grow throughout the world. Their name is derived from the presence of stinging hairs on their leaves and stems which when touched inject formic acid and histamine into the skin and cause urticaria (or inflammation). Nettles have been widely used as food, and in medicines, cosmetics, and clothing.

Nettles are a rich source of trace elements, absorbing and accumulating them. They contain formic acid and the neurotransmitters acetylcholine, 5-hydroxy tryptamine, and histamine which are responsible for the sting. These constituents are thought to endow nettles with their anti-arthritic, antirheumatic and expectorant properties.

Because of their rich nutritional content, nettles have traditionally been given to anemic, exhausted, debilitated or recuperating individuals as soups or teas. The stinging properties are lost when the plant is cooked. Nettles also have been traditionally used as an important hair and skin tonic. The high quantity of silicon has made nettles highly useful in stimulating hair growth, improving the condition of the hair and skin and treating dandruff. Nettles have been used both internally and externally to treat eczema. Nettle juice has been used as an astringent or styptic to stop bleeding and to treat wounds.

The best known use of nettles is in the treatment of gout and other rheumatic conditions. A decoction of the leaves or the expressed juice has been shown to mobilize uric acid from the joints and eliminate it through the kidneys. Recently, a randomized, double blind, clinical trial has shown the usefulness of nettles in the treatment of allergic rhinitis or hayfever.

TRADITIONAL AND OTHER THERAPEUTIC USES

- treats gout, arthritis, tendinitis, sciatica, and lumbago
- treats eczema
- halts hair loss and deterioration
- treats allergic rhinitis, hayfever, sinusitis, sinus congestion
- aids recovery from anemia and exhaustion
- acts as an astringent and styptic in wound healing
- treats profuse menstruation
- treats benign prostatic hypertrophy
- reduces inflammation
- acts as a mild diuretic
- encourages lactation
- lowers blood sugar

NONI
(Morinda citrifolia)

ORIGIN
    Hawaii

PART OF PLANT USED
    Fruit

DESCRIPTION
    "Noni" or Morinda citrifolia grows in mountainous areas of Hawaii, and has been used for centuries by the traditional medicine men, or kahunas, to treat a wide variety of health concerns. An ancient plant whose healing properties helped form the foundation of traditional Hawaiian healing arts, it has been shown to be effective against several bacteria including E. coli. A 1992 study showed that noni has unique immune-stimulating effects. A 1993 study revealed similar results for this important plant. A 1990 study proved Morinda citrifolia to also have analgesic properties.

    The noni plant and its fruit have an extremely foul odor and taste. A process has been developed to remove them while preserving noni's healing qualities.

TRADITIONAL AND OTHER THERAPEUTIC USES
- joint pain and general pain relief
- immune system problems
- inflammation
- cellular regeneration

OLIVE LEAF
(Olea europaea L.)

ORIGIN
Mediterranean

PART OF PLANT USED
Leaf

DESCRIPTION
Around 1855, medical information began to appear describing the potential cure of the protozoa-caused disease, malaria, by drinking a bitter tea brewed from olive leaves. Doctors reported that their patients improved as a result of these trials against malaria. Further into the nineteenth century, a phenolin compound, oleuropein, was isolated from the olive leaf. It is considered to be a source of the olive tree's powerful disease resistant properties. Laboratory analysis shows oleuropein to be a bitter glucoside present in the pulp of live fruits. Glucosides are one of a group of compounds which contain the cyclic form of glucose, in which an alkyl or aryl group has replaced the hydrogen of the hemiacetal hydroxyl. According to botanists, oleuropein, which is present throughout the olive tree (in its wood, fruits, leaves, roots, and bark) helps to protect it against insects and bacteria.

By 1969, more molecular analysis had taken place and researchers uncovered the main antiviral ingredient present in oleuropein. Inhibiting the growth of every virus that it was tested against, this ingredient was identified as the calcium salt of elenolic acid, calcium elenolate. Viruses, which were killed by the substance, were the coxsackie virus, parainfluenza 3 virus, herpes virus, the encephalomyocarditis virus, Newcastle disease virus, polio virus, and the Sindbis virus.

Pure calcium elenolate is obtained after mild acid hydrolysis from the aqueous extracts of various parts of the olive plant. The calcium salt was of hydrolysates and this crystalline substance is then powdered for creating tablets or capsules of the virucidal nutritional supplement. Olive leaf extract is a viable nutritional supplement for virucidal and other antimicrobial uses.

TRADITIONAL AND OTHER THERAPEUTIC USES

- interferes with processes necessary for the production of certain viruses by inactivating viruses or by preventing virus shedding, budding, or assembly at the cell membrane
- penetrates infected host cells and irrevocably inhibits viral replication
- stimulates phagocytosis as an immune system response

PASSION FLOWER
(Passiflora incarnata)

ORIGIN
North and South America, Europe

PART OF PLANT USED
Dried above ground parts, gathered during the fruiting season

DESCRIPTION
Passion flower is a woody vine with flowers which reminded early Jesuit travellers of the passion or suffering of Christ. The plant produces a small berry-like fruit called granadilla or water lemon.

Passion flower contains glycosides (containing alkaloids) and flavonoids. Low levels of serotonin have been identified which may help explain the use of passion flower as a natural calmative, mood shifter, and aid to concentration. Another compound called "maltol" has been shown to have mild sedative properties. The harmane alkaloids have been shown to be spasmolytic toward smooth muscle and to lower blood pressure by expanding heart coronary vessels.

For the past 200 years, passion flower has been used to tranquilize and settle edgy nerves. Passion flower induces sleep without causing confusion upon awakening. Passion flower has been used by women to calm nerves and induce relaxation during the periods of hormonal adjustment found during menses and menopause.

TRADITIONAL AND OTHER THERAPEUTIC USES
- a mild sedative, it combats sleeplessness
- useful in calming nervous and high-strung, hyperactive children

- treats cardiovascular "neurosis"
- improves concentration
- beneficial for hormonal adjustment, menses, and menopausal problems
- treats bronchial asthma
- combats hemorrhoidal inflammation
- acts as an antispasmodic
- acts as an analgesic and anticonvulsant

TOXICITY, CAUTIONS AND CONTRAINDICATIONS

No known toxicity when using standardized whole plant extracts.

PASSION VINE
(Passiflora incarnata)

ORIGIN
Southern North America

DESCRIPTION
Passiflora incarnata, the plant often used to induce sleep, is one of the northern-most of the passion vines. Whereas most of them are indigenous to tropical America, the "maypop," as it is known, ranges as far north as Virginia. All of the members of the passion vine family contain chemicals with relaxing properties to some degree, and the maypop is the best of them for an overactive mind when it comes time to fall asleep.

Passion vine has a depressing effect on the central nervous system, which means that it slows the action of the nerves. This is why the herb is helpful in cases of insomnia and muscular spasms. It is one of the best botanic drugs for hyperactivity of the nerves and any condition that results from it, including severe spasms, epilepsy, chorea, tetanus, hysteria, and persistent hiccup.

Passion vine is anti-spasmodic, hypnotic, and tonic. It quiets nervous irritation and promotes sleep, tones up the sympathetic nervous system, and improves circulation and nutrition. Passion vine is of use in some cases of spasm in children, and it may be employed as a nervine at the menstrual period. Insomnia resulting from fevers, particularly from some forms of typhoid, can be helped by this herb.

At a certain point, a person needs to sleep even though his or her nervous system is so agitated that sleep without an aid is impossible. The Eclectics felt that maypop was perfect for inducing sleep in this circumstance. It will gently slow the system down so that the person can drift off to sleep without fear of a hangover the next day. This cannot be said of sleeping pills, thus making passion vine superior.

For people with chronic insomnia, taking drugs on a regular basis to induce sleep is inappropriate, whether they are pharmaceutical or herbal preparations. If one suffers from insomnia more than two nights a week, he or she has a definite problem and it may require professional help to sort it out. Though there are exceptions to this rule, generally speaking, if one cannot sleep at night, he or she is doing something wrong during the day. It could be too much intake of caffeine, or it could be living life at too fast a pace. In either case, behavior needs to change. It is not acceptable to be dependent on any preparation to regularly fall asleep.

PAU D'ARCO
(Tabebuia avellanedae)

ORIGIN
South America

PART OF PLANT USED
Inner bark

DESCRIPTION
Pau d'arco is an ancient Brazilian remedy taken from the inner bark of lapacho trees of the species, purple Tabebuia avellanedae. The bark is boiled for tea, the form in which it seems to be most effective.

It is used in some hospitals in South America with great success on cancer patients. A powerful antibiotic with virus-killing properties, pau d'arco is also known as Taheebo, its Indian name.

Pau d'arco is high in iron, which aids in the proper assimilation of nutrients and the elimination of wastes. It is a detoxifier. Pau d'arco is said to contain compounds, which seem to attack the cause of disease, putting the body in a defensive state to give it the energy needed to help resist disease.

A bitter herb that contains natural antibacterial and antifungal agents, it has a healing effect and cleanses the blood. It has been used for smoker's cough, warts, all types of infection, diabetes, ulcers, rheumatism, allergies, tumors, AIDS and liver disease. Pau d'arco is especially good for pain related to cancer.

People with Candida have found pau d'arco tea to be beneficial in controlling the growth. Traditional uses have included coughs, bacterial infections, fungal infections, allergies, ulcers, and rheumatism.

TRADITIONAL AND OTHER THERAPEUTIC USES

- treats anemia
- improves appetite
- purifies the blood, acting as a general cleanser
- fights cancer, including leukemia
- effectively treats insomnia
- treats nervous disorders
- alleviates pain
- improves conditions of the prostate gland and aids the kidneys
- treats rheumatism
- kills ringworm
- treats skin problems
- treats ulcers

TOXICITY, CAUTIONS AND CONTRAINDICATIONS

No known toxicity.

PEPPERMINT
(Mentha piperita)

ORIGIN
Mediterranean

PART OF PLANT USED
Leaves

DESCRIPTION
"Mint" is the name for any number of plants belonging to the Labiatae family, all of which produce the characteristic minty scent when the leaves are crushed. The most medicinal of the mints is Mentha piperita, peppermint. When looking for mint to use for the stomach, it is best to specify peppermint.

Originally native to the Mediterranean region, the plant can be found all over the planet due to its voracious growing habits and its usefulness to humankind. Though stomach abuse is currently at an all-time high, poor eating habits have been a problem throughout human history. Mint's medicinal use predates the Bible. The ancient Romans carried it with them wherever they colonized. To this day, Arabs brew it into tea and chop it into salads. Indians include it in chutney recipes. The British make its juice into jellies to be served with heavy meat dishes. Germans concoct it into schnapps as an after dinner drink. In all these cases, the motive for including mint in the diet is to improve digestion and avoid indigestion.

TRADITIONAL AND OTHER THERAPEUTIC USES
- treats indigestion and facilitates digestion by stimulating the secretion of bile and digestive juices
- improves the stomach's functioning

- carminative (antigas)
- anti-inflammatory
- antispasmodic/muscle relaxant
- antiemetic (preventing vomiting)
- nervine (soothing to the nerves)
- antimicrobial
- analgesic, especially effective for nerves in the stomach

TOXICITY, CAUTIONS AND CONTRAINDICATIONS

No known toxicity.

PSYLLIUM
(Plantago ovata)

ORIGIN
India

PART OF PLANT USED
Seed hulls

DESCRIPTION

Dietary fiber, formerly unrecognized for its health benefits, has received much attention as of late. It is widely accepted as playing a significant role in reducing total blood cholesterol, thereby decreasing the risk of coronary heart disease, and in helping to alleviate numerous bowel disorders.

Dietary fiber can be divided into two basic categories, soluble and insoluble. Soluble fiber dissolves in water, and insoluble fiber, as the term describes, does not. Both types of fiber provide bulk in the large intestine and encourage bowel regularity. However, there are, it seems, some quite important additional benefits to be derived from the effects of soluble fiber on the digestive system and on cholesterol.

Psyllium is a natural, water-soluble, gel-producing fiber, which is extracted from the husks of blond psyllium seeds (Plantago ovata). Psyllium is a member of a class of soluble fibers referred to as mucilages. Mucilages, which retain water, tend to be rather thick and jelly-like in nature. Also in the mucilage family is guar gum, an ingredient in most beans. It is used as a stabilizing and thickening agent in many salad dressings, soups, lotions, and creams. Other commonly used dietary fibers include wheat bran, which is, for the most part, insoluble and classified as a cellulose fiber. Also widely used are oat bran, a hemicellulose fiber, and apple pectin, both of which are water-soluble.

The water-soluble fibers such as psyllium, oat bran, apple pectin, and guar gum have demonstrated an ability to lower blood cholesterol levels. Therories concerning how this is accomplished include the ability of water-soluble fiber to increase the excretion of cholesterol through the bowel, to inhibit its synthesis in the liver, and to bind to and absorb bile acids in the intestine. The water insoluble fibers, wheat bran, for example, have not exhibited the same success in lowering cholesterol as have water-soluble fibers.

It is clear that supplementing your diet with a water-soluble fiber such as psyllium can provide many benefits. Whether you suffer from occasional bouts of constipation or diarrhea, diabetes, food cravings, high cholesterol or simply want to "clean" your colon, psyllium may be just what you need.

TRADITIONAL AND OTHER THERAPEUTIC USES

- lowers cholesterol; a well tolerated therapy or adjunct for mild to moderate hypercholesterolemia.
- combats digestive complaints such as constipation, diarrhea, diverticular disease and colitis
- utilized as part of many colon "cleansing" programs and even in the prevention of colon cancer
- lowers the incidence of hemorrhoids and thrombosis
- works to rid the colon of toxic substances, including heavy metals
- encourages the growth of healthful, "friendly" intestinal bacteria such as Lactobacillus acidophilus
- slows down emptying food from the stomach, decreasing hunger when taken with meals
- stimulates pancreatic enzyme secretion

TOXICITY, CAUTIONS AND CONTRAINDICATIONS

There has been no reported toxicity, however, there are people who have a low tolerance for fiber in their diets. In such cases, psyllium and other fibers can cause intestinal irritability with gas, bloating, and pain. Some medications (e.g. narcotics) may decrease intestinal motility and "bulk laxitives" should not be used unless cleared by the prescribing physician. There have also been cases of people having allergic reactions to psyllium, although these have been extremely rare. A word of caution: if taking a drug to control cholesterol level, one would be well advised to consult with his or her physician before attempting to lower the dosage or discontinue its use.

PYGEUM
(Pygeum africanum)

ORIGIN
Southern and central Africa, Madagascar

PART OF PLANT USED
Bark

DESCRIPTION

Pygeum is a large evergreen tree growing in the high plateaus of southern Africa. Traditionally the bark of the tree was collected and powdered, then drunk as a tea for genitourinary complaints. Recently numerous clinical trials have demonstrated the usefulness of a standardized extract of pygeum for enlargement of the prostate, particularly benign prostatic hypertrophy (BPH).

Pygeum contains a number of active components including phytosterols such as beta-sitosterol; pentacyclic triterpenoids, such as ursolic and oleanic acids; and ferulic esters of fatty alcohols, particularly fatty esters of docosanol and tetracosanol. The phytosterols, particularly beta-sitosterol, are found in numerous plants and are anti-inflammatory, inhibiting the synthesis of prostaglandins. Beta-sitosterol has been shown to be useful in cases of BPH by helping to reduce the normally elevated levels of prostaglandins in these patients. The elimination of the excess blood and vessel congestion can help reduce the size of prostate adenomas. The pentacyclic triterpenoids also help inhibit inflammation by blocking enzymatic activity. They are effective anti-edema agents and also help increase the integrity of small veins and capillaries. The third active group, the ferulic esters of long-chain fatty acids, act by inhibiting the absorption and metabolism of cholesterol. BPH and other cases of enlargement of the prostate are often associated with abnormally high levels of cholesterol.

Pygeum has been studied in numerous double blind clinical trials and found to be effective in treating a wide range of prostatic hyperplasias. Efficacy was determined by measuring the effects of extracts of pygeum on numerous parameters, including dysuria, nocturia, frequent urination, abnormal heaviness, residual urine, prostate volume and peak flow. Consumption of pygeum extract resulted in significant amelioration of symptoms, reduction of prostate size, and clearance of bladder neck urethral obstruction.

TRADITIONAL AND OTHER THERAPEUTIC USES
- prostatitis
- benign prostatic hyperrophy (BPH)
- urinary retention
- incontinence
- polyuria or frequent urination
- dysuria
- painful urination
- nocturia (nocturnal urination)
- possibly helpful in cancers of the prostate
- adenomatous fibrosclerosis

RHODIOLA ROSEA

DESCRIPTION

Rhodiola rosea (also known as Arctic root or golden root) is a member of the family Crassulaceae, a family of plants native to the arctic regions of eastern Siberia. It grows at altitudes of 11,000 to 18,000 feet above sea level. As an herb, it grows approximately 2 1/2 feet high and has yellow flowers whose smell is similar to attar of roses, thus imparting its name.

Rhodiola would be classified as an adaptogen, meaning that it has a nonspecific ability to assist the body to withstand stress and maintain normalcy even when threatened with pathological conditions. As such, it is similar to a number of other herbs classified as adaptogens including Siberian ginseng, reishi mushroom, ginseng, cordyceps and ashwagandha. In Siberia it is said, "those who drink rhodiola tea regularly will live more than 100 years.". Chinese emperors, always looking for the secret to long life and immortality, sent expeditions into Siberia to collect and bring back the plant. Being one of the most popular medicinal herbs of middle Asia, for many years Rhodiola was illegally transported across the Russian border to China. In Siberia it was taken regularly especially during the cold and wet winters to prevent sickness. In Mongolia it was used for the treatment of tuberculosis and cancer.

Formerly regarded as a scarce plant, researchers from Tomsk State University found significant stands of this valuable herb growing wild in Siberia at elevations of 5000 to 9000 feet above sea level. Subsequent research has substantiated high life giving biological activity with no toxicity. For the treatment of depression, extracts of rhodiola, rosavin and salidroside used in animal studies seem to enhance the transport of serotonin precursors, tryptophan, and 5-hydroxytryptophan, into the brain. Serotonin is a widely studied brain neurotransmitter that is involved in many functions including smooth muscle contraction, pain perception, and temperature, appetite, blood pressure, and respiratory regulation. Proper serotonin levels can impart a sense of contentment and mental ease. Either too much or too little serotonin has been linked to various abnormal mental states such as clinical depression. Thus rhodiola has been used by Russian scientists alone or in combination with antidepressants to boost one's mental state, a boon in countries and especially during seasons when one is deprived of adequate sunlight over prolonged periods. This leads to a condition known as Seasonal Affective Disorder (SAD) common to Northern European countries.

Rhodiola has also been shown to be effective for cardiac problems caused or aggravated by stress. Its action for these conditions is in its ability to decrease the amount of catecholamines and corticosteroids released by the adrenal glands during stress. The abnormal presence of these stress hormones will subsequently raise blood pressure, cholesterol, and potassium levels, increasing the risk of heart disease. Rhodiola has been found to decrease harmful blood lipids and thus decrease the risk of heart disease. It also decreases the amount of cyclic-AMP (c-AMP) released into cardiac cells. Cyclic AMP is related to ATP (adenosine triphosphate), the body's primary energy molecule. C-AMP assists in the uptake of extracellular calcium into the heart muscle, promoting a greater potential for heart muscle contraction and regulating the heartbeat, thus helping counteract heart arrhythmias.

As an adaptogen, rhodiola both stimulates and protects the immune system by reinstating homeostasis (metabolic balance) in the body. It also increases natural killer (NK) cells in the stomach and spleen. This action may be due to its ability to normalize hormones by modulating the release of glucocorticoids into the body.

Rhodiola has potent antioxidant properties. By limiting the adverse effects of free radical damage, it is able to combat diseases associated with aging. The presence of free radicals is associated with cell mutagenicity, the immediate cause of cancer. Russian researchers found that oral administration of rhodiola inhibited tumor growth in rats 39 percent and decreased metastasis by 50 percent. It improved urinary tissue and immunity in patients suffering with bladder cancer. In other studies with various types of cancer, including adenocarcinoma (cancer of glandular tissue such as breast cancer) and lung carcinoma, the use of extracts of rhodiola rosea resulted in significant increased survival rate.

Rhodiola is often used by athletes to improve performance. While the mechanism is not completely understood, rhodiola seems to improve the body's muscle-to-fat ratio and increases the hemoglobin concentration and erythrocyte count in the blood.

Many other benefits from the use of Rhodiola have been found. These include improved hearing, suppressed progression of pyorrhea in burns, regulation of blood sugar levels in those with diabetes, and protection of the liver from environmental toxins.

Nearly 200 different rhodiola species have been identified. Only 14 have been subjected to biochemical study and it has been found that the chemical composition and pharmacological activity of rhodiola is definitely species related. In general, rhodiola contains phenylpropanoids, proanthocyanidins and flavonoids. The most uniquely active chemical constituents are the phenylpropanoids, rosavin (the most active), rosin, rosarin, rhodiolin, salidroside, and its aglycon, p-tyrosol. Only Rhodiola rosea contains rosavin, rosin and rosarin.

In summary, Rhodiola rosea counteracts the effects of stress that ultimately underlies the evolution of many diseases.

TRADITIONAL AND OTHER THERAPEUTIC USES

- stress
- depression

TOXICITY, CAUTIONS AND CONTRAINDICATIONS

None.

SAW PALMETTO
(Serenoa serrulata)

ORIGIN
North American Atlantic coast

PART OF PLANT USED
Berries

DESCRIPTION
Saw palmetto is a small palm tree with large leaves and large deep red-black berries. The berries were used by native North Americans as a general tonic to nourish the body and encourage appetite and normal weight gain. The berries were also used in the treatment of genitourinary tract problems including enuresis and nocturia. Recent clinical trials have shown that saw palmetto berries are helpful in the treatment of benign prostatic hyperplasia.

The berries of saw palmetto contain an oil with a variety of fatty acids and phytosterols. The fat-soluble extract of saw palmetto berries has been shown to inhibit the conversion of testosterone to dihydrotestosterone (DHT), which is thought to be responsible for the enlargement of the prostate. In addition, saw palmetto extract inhibits the binding of DHT to receptors, thus blocking DHT's action and promoting the breakdown of the potent compound.

The native North Americans used saw palmetto berries as a remedy for atrophy of the testes, impotence, inflammation of the prostate, and low libido in men. The berries have been recommended for infertility, painful periods, and lactation in women. The berries also have a traditional use as a tonic and expectorant for mucous membranes, particularly the bronchial passages.

TRADITIONAL AND OTHER THERAPEUTIC USES

- urinary tract disorders, nocturia, and enuresis
- benign prostatic hypertrophy and prostate inflammation
- impotence and low libido
- atrophy of the testes
- infertility in women (a tonic for ovarian function)
- used to increase lactation
- painful menstrual periods
- expectorant and inhalant for bronchitis, asthma, and colds
- tonic for mucous membranes
- mildly sedative to the nervous system
- anti-inflammatory
- appetite stimulant, improving digestion
- thyroid deficiency

TOXICITY, CAUTIONS AND CONTRAINDICATIONS

No reported toxicity

ST. JOHN'S WORT
(Hypericum perforatum)

ORIGIN
Worldwide

PART OF PLANT USED
Aerial parts

DESCRIPTION

St. John's wort is a perennial with regular flowers, which bloom from June until September. The plant was believed, from the time of the ancient Greeks until the Middle Ages, to ward off witchcraft and evil spirits, driving out devils. Considered a noxious weed by farmers due to its photosensitizing effect on livestock, St. John's wort has nevertheless been used by humans for centuries for a wide variety of ailments, including nervous disorders, depression, neuralgia, wounds, burns, and kidney problems. It is also valued for its antibacterial and anti-inflammatory actions. Recently, a great deal of attention has been placed on the herb because of its two main active ingredients, hypericin and pseudohypericin, which have been shown to inhibit the AIDS virus.

St. John's wort contains a variety of active ingredients including dianthrone derivatives (hypericin and pseudohypericin), xanthrones, flavonoids and tannins. Xanthrones and hypericin have been shown to have monoamine-oxidase (MAO) inhibiting activity. A standard treatment for depression uses MAO inhibitors to retard the breakdown of central nervous system neurotransmitters such as norepinephrine and serotonin, thus increasing concentration. A clinical trial involving standardized hypericin extract showed improvement in depressive symptoms, including anxiety, apathy, insomnia and feelings of worthlessness. The flavonoids and possibly other agents have wound healing and anti-inflammatory activities. Most current research has focused on the antiviral activity of the anthrowuinones, hypericin and pseudohypericin. Hypericin is a photodynamic red pigment whose antiviral activity is substantially enhanced by exposure to light. The mechanism is thought to involve the production of oxygen free radicals, which can damage the viral envelope. Non-enveloped viruses such as polio or adenovirus are unaffected by hypericin. Human studies involved taking high doses of hypericin (10 mg) extracted from St. John's wort.

St. John's wort has been used for centuries to calm the nerves and treat depression. A red oil made from macerating the flowers in vegetable oil has been used to dress wounds, heal deep cuts, soothe burns and ease the pain of neuralgias. Taken internally, the oil has been used for ulcers and gastritis. An infusion of the herb has also been used as an expectorant for bronchitis, as a diuretic for the kidneys, and as an easing agent for menstrual cramps.

TRADITIONAL AND OTHER THERAPEUTIC USES
- depression, psychological illness, mania, fear, nervous disorders, and hysteria
- sedative
- wound and burn healing (applied externally)
- antibacterial and antiviral, with possible benefit against AIDS
- bed-wetting and childhood nightmares
- gastric ulcers
- inflammation
- genitourinary troubles
- diuretic
- menstrual cramps

TOXICITY, CAUTIONS AND CONTRAINDICATIONS

Consumption of hypericin may render the skin photosensitive. Care should be taken during exposure to sunlight. Avoid excessive exposure to sunlight, tanning lights or UV sources.

SUMA
(Pffafia paniculata)

ORIGIN
Brazil

PART OF PLANT USED
Roots

DESCRIPTION
Suma is one of the most highly regarded herbs from South America and is native to the mid-Atlantic rain forest region of Brazil. The plant consists of a ground-covering vine with an intricate and deep root structure. The root of Pfaffia paniculata has been used by the indigenous people for three centuries. Suma has been considered to be a true adaptogen as well as a remedy for diabetes, ulcers, wounds, and cancer. Recently, suma extracts have been used for muscle building and the treatment of chronic fatigue syndrome (CFS). Suma is known as an adaptogen because of its ability to enhance endurance and vitality. Adaptogens such as suma and ginseng help the body achieve a physiological balance resulting in improved resistance to infections and increased resistance to stress.

Among the many ingredients found in suma, the most notable is ecdysterone. Also known as B-ecdysterone, this phytosterol or plant hormone is very similar in use to alpha-ecdysone, an insect molting hormone. Suma is considered to be one of the richest sources of B-ecdysterone. Ecdysones and plant sterols in general, have been the focus of a great deal of research all over the world for their anabolic effects and a variety of applications. Other phytosterols found in suma include beta-sitosterol, polypodine B, and stigmasterol. There are many other nutrients found in this plant, including a broad spectrum of vitamins, minerals and amino acids. Allantoin, a cell-building compound, and trace amounts of germanium are also found. Other active constituents include six unique saponins called pfaffosides, as well as pfaffic acid.

TRADITIONAL AND OTHER THERAPEUTIC USES

- can increase endurance
- enhances stress resistance and immune function
- decreases inflammation
- accelerates wound and fracture healing
- anti-inflammatory
- anabolic, increasing protein levels
- analgesic
- decreases cholesterol levels
- several anticancer effects of the constituents of the root have recently been discovered

TOXICITY, CAUTIONS AND CONTRAINDICATIONS

Suma shows very low toxicity and does not appear to cause adverse reactions. Because of suma's natural hormones, it should not be taken during pregnancy.

THYME
(Thymus vulgaris)

ORIGIN
Mediterranean

PART OF PLANT USED
Leaves

DESCRIPTION

Thyme is native to the Mediterranean region. Thanks to its medicinal and culinary virtues, it can now be found wherever the winters are mild. This low-growing, creeping plant is thought to have spread from its original range well into northern Europe along with the conquering Roman soldiers. There is some controversy as to how the plant got its scientific name, 'Thymus.' Some say it comes from the Greek word, 'thumos,' or courage, which the plant was believed to convey to the person who drank a tea made of it. Others say it comes from a similar Greek word which means "to fumigate," a use to which the plant was also put in ancient days.

In English herbalism, thyme was the traditional cure for all manner of ills affecting the lungs. Culpepper called thyme "a noble strengthener of the lungs, as notable are as grows, nor is there a better remedy growing for whooping cough. It purgeth the body of phlegm and is an excellent remedy for shortness of breath. It is so harmless you need not fear the use of it." His statement is reiterated by most of the classic English herbalists. In traditional European herbalism, thyme was used to treat respiratory infections, laryngitis, tonsillitis, sore throats, irritable coughs, bronchitis, whooping cough, asthma and catarrhal coughs. Even the U.S. Food and Drug Administration agrees with Culpepper as to the plant's harmlessness, rating it "generally recognized as food safe."

The actions of the plant include carminative, antimicrobial, antispasmodic, expectorant, astringent, and anthelmintic. Chemicals contained in the herb responsible for these actions include a volatile oil composed of thymol, carvacrol, cineole, borneol, geraniol, linalool, bornyl and linalyl acetate, thymol methyl ether and alpha pinene. Its flavonoids include apigenin, luteolin, thymonin, and naringenin. Also included are labiatic acid, caffeic acid and tannins.

One of the plant's chief medicinally active ingredients is the crystalline phenol called thymol. First isolated in 1720, it was later studied and found to be a rather amazing substance, powerfully antiseptic, both internally and externally. To make matters better, it is an effective analgesic or painkiller. Early on, thymol was shown to kill bacteria on contact and therefore is found in surgical dressings and disinfectants for everything from wounds to surgical theaters. Thymol and the plant that contains it were used to kill bacteria, and this tradition continues.

Thyme was used by the Greeks to fumigate, and some say it was used specifically to fumigate sickrooms. Though modern physicians tend to discredit herbal medicine, the ancient custom of burning thyme in a sickroom would have been efficacious. Thymol released into the air by burning the herb would make the patient's attendants less likely to contract his illness if it were bacterial in nature. Sage and rosemary, close relations of thyme, were also burned in sickrooms, jails, churches and public halls to stop the spread of diseases such as "jail fever." These plants were being used as bactericides long before bacteria had even been discovered.

TRADITIONAL AND OTHER THERAPEUTIC USES

- stimulates the movement of mucus out of the chest cavity
- provides antimicrobial chemicals to kill infection (antifungal and antibacterial)
- acts as an antispasmodic, which helps with the pain associated with coughing
- gargle for laryngitis, tonsillitis and sore throats in general
- expectorant

TRIBULUS TERRESTRIS
(Puncture Vine)

DESCRIPTION

Tribulus terrestris is an herb commonly known as "Puncture Vine" or Caltrop fruit, grown in various parts of the world and used medicinally for its virilizing effects. Studies have shown a better than 50% increase in testosterone levels when taking the Tribulus terrestris herb.

The Chemical Pharmaceutical Institute in Sofia, Bulgaria conducted clinical studies on Tribulus, which showed improved reproductive functions, including increased sperm production and testosterone levels in men. When scientists began studying the remarkable curative power of Tribulus terrestris, they discovered that it significantly elevates the level of several hormones, including testosterone, Luteinizing Hormone (LH is a gonad stimulating hormone produced by the pituitary gland), Follicle Stimulating Hormone (FSH), and estradiol. A significant benefit of Tribulus is the stimulation of hormone production to a balanced level, without over stimulating the secretion of hormones.

Tribulus terrestris has been used for centuries in Europe for hormone insufficiency in men. Chinese herbalists have been using it in the treatment of liver, kidney and urinary tract disease, as well as all types of skin disorders.

The fruit and root of Tribulus contain pharmacologically important metabolites like phytosteroids, flavonoids, alkaloids and glycosides. These active components have a stimulating effect on the immune and reproductive systems, with improved muscle building, stamina and endurance. Other positive changes observed in a number of cases were a reduction in cholesterol and enhanced mood and well-being. Tribulus also exhibits a mild diuretic effect.

The liver is a major synthesizer of hormones. They are synthesized from cholesterol, so an herb such as Tribulus that has a stimulating effect on the liver, will have a major influence on cholesterol and other products of the liver. Tribulus' role as a liver tonic is very important, breaking down the cholesterol and fats that inhibit healthy liver function. The cholesterol and fats are converted to hormones and there is a resulting increased performance and stamina. This role of improving liver function, stamina and endurance is particularly beneficial to athletes and bodybuilders.

No adverse effects to the central nervous or cardiovascular systems were noted in any of the clinical studies. No toxicity and no deviations in blood count occurred. No known negative effects presently exist when Tribulus is used as a dietary supplement.

The increase in testosterone levels by Tribulus will promote protein synthesis and positive nitrogen balance, as well as faster recuperation and recovery from muscular stress. Tribulus therefore has a positive effect on strength and stamina.

TRADITIONAL AND OTHER THERAPEUTIC USES

- improves stamina
- increases testosterone levels
- beneficial to athletes and bodybuilders

TOXICITY, CAUTIONS AND CONTRADICTIONS

None noted.

TURMERIC
(Curcuma longa)

ORIGIN
India

PART OF PLANT USED
Rhizome

DESCRIPTION

Turmeric has long been considered an essential flavoring spice of Indian and other ethnic cuisines. Turmeric provides the typical yellow color of many curry dishes and helps to render food more digestible. Turmeric, along with other curry herbs, has several physiologic activities, including the inhibition of platelet aggregation, antibiotic effects, anticholesterol action, and fibrinolytic activity.

Many studies on turmeric have revealed that the herb contains cholagogue-type substances, which increase the secretion of bile. Principal among these substances is curcumin which posesses liver protective activity, detoxifying dangerous carcinogens, stimulating the gall bladder and acting as a free radical scavenger. Curcumin has cholekinetic activity (bile duct stimulation). It has been suggested that tumeric lowers blood cholesterol through these various choleric effects. Turmeric's effects on weight loss may also be mediated through curcumin's catabolic and metabolic activities on fats. Studies have also revealed that curcumin has anti-inflammatory properties, inhibiting platelet aggregation and cyclooxgenase and lipoxygenase enzymes which catalyze the formation of inflammatory prostaglandins and other molecules. Curcumin requires the presence of the adrenal glands to have this non-steroidal anti-inflammatory activity.

TRADITIONAL AND OTHER THERAPEUTIC USES

- used in folk medicine to treat arthritis
- anti-inflammatory
- cholagogue that stimulates digestion, used for indigestion
- protects the liver (heptoprotective) and treats liver disease such as hepatitis
- gall bladder and bile duct diseases
- used in treating obesity
- has strong antibacterial and antifungal properties
- lowers blood cholesterol
- possible cancer preventive

TOXICITY, CAUTIONS AND CONTRAINDICATIONS

No known toxicity. Large doses are not recommended in cases of painful gallstones, obstructive jaundice, acute bilious colic or extremely toxic liver disorders.

UVA URSI
(Arctostaphylos uva–ursi)

ORIGIN
Northern United States and Europe

PART OF PLANT USED
Leaves

DESCRIPTION
Uva ursi is a small perennial evergreen shrub. White flowers tinged with red bloom from June to September, which are followed by small edible red berries. Uva ursi leaf is widely used as a diuretic, astringent, and antiseptic. Folk medicine around the world has recommended uva ursi for nephritis, kidney stones and chronic cystitis. The herb has also been used as a general tonic for weakened kidneys, liver or pancreas.

Uva ursi contains a high concentration of arbutin, an antiseptic phenolic glycoside having diuretic and urinary antiseptic action. They relieve pain from bladder stones, cystitis, nephritis and kidney stones. Arbutin is converted in the body to glucose and hydroquinones, which has antiseptic and disinfecting properties if the urine is alkaline. The hydroquinone will turn the urine green. Uva ursi also contains allantion, which is known for its soothing and tissue-repairing properties.

TOXICITY, CAUTIONS AND CONTRAINDICATIONS
The following cautions should be observed. Uva ursi requires an alkaline pH to work. It is contraindicated as a urinary disinfectant under conditions of acid urine (urine can be made alkaline by ingesting a heaping teaspoon of

bicarbonate of soda). Uva ursi is contraindicated as a diuretic or flushing agent in acute cystitis. It can induce gastric irritation if overused due to the tannin concentration. Uva ursi should not be used during pregnancy.

VALERIAN
(Valeriana officinalis)

ORIGIN
Europe

PARTS OF PLANT USED
Rhizome, root-stock

DESCRIPTION

Since ancient Greek times, valerian root has been valued as an antispasmodic and sleep aid. The first known records reported its use in the treatment of epilepsy. Today, valerian is widely used throughout Europe as a mild sedative and sleep aid for insomnia. It is also used as a balancing agent for hyperexcitability and exhaustion, calming one and stimulating the other.

The sedative effects of valerian root are attributed to the valepotriates, a group of unstable esters whose degradation products also possess sedative activity. Other components, particularly those of the pungent essential oil, the valerenic and isovaleric acids, have sedative and central nervous system (CNS) depressant activity. Researchers have also established that the valepotriates and the other components of valerian possess relaxing and spasmolytic effects on smooth muscle. A mechanism has been proposed for the central nervous system effects involving the metabolism of gamma-aminobutyric acid (GABA) in the brain. Valerian appears the most effective when all its constituents are present. The different activities of valerian appear to be due to a complex mixture of substances.

Numerous clinical trials have been performed with valerian root and have found both subjective and objective reductions in emotional tension and improvements in sleep quality without producing a hangover type effect the next morning.

TRADITIONAL AND OTHER THERAPEUTIC USES

- insomnia, especially due to nervous exhaustion
- motoric restlessness or vegetative dysfunction
- headaches
- anxiety and nervous tension
- palpitations
- high blood pressure
- antispasmodic
- nervous dyspepsia and stomach cramps
- spastic or irritable bowel
- menstrual cramps
- dandruff
- epilepsy
- childhood behavioral disorders and learning disabilities

TOXICITY, CAUTIONS AND CONTRAINDICATIONS

No known toxicity. High doses (5 g root/day) can lead to minor withdrawal symptoms upon discontinuance if taken over a long period of time. Avoid large doses and prolonged use.

WHEATGRASS

ORIGIN
Worldwide

PART OF PLANT USED
Juice of sprouted kernels

DESCRIPTION
One of the so-called "green foods," wheatgrass is valued as a great source of nutrients. It is wheatgrass's chlorophyll that is perhaps its most valuable asset. The green pigment has been shown in studies to have cleansing, detoxifying, and healing effects on the body.

Wheatgrass is sprouted wheat kernels, harvested when the sprouts are just a week old. Because its fibers are indigestible for humans, it must be liquefied in a juicer before it can be consumed. One can drink the juice straight or in a more palatable mixture with other juices. It is best to consume the beverage in small quantities, not to exceed four fluid ounces (118 ml) per day. Due to its strong cleansing properties, excessive consumption of the juice can cause nausea or stomach upset. It also is converted into tablet form.

Whether taken as juice or tablets, wheatgrass is said to cleanse the blood, organs, and gastrointestinal tract. It is also recommended as a way to stimulate metabolism and enzyme systems. It reportedly stimulates and normalizes the thyroid gland, which may be helpful in correcting obesity and indigestion.

Wheatgrass contains a variety of vitamins, minerals, amino acids and enzymes. It has an abundance of alkaline minerals, claimed to help reduce blood acidity. It is a potent source of vitamins A, B, C, and E. Minerals include calcium, iron, sodium, potassium, magnesium, and a variety of trace minerals such as selenium and zinc.

While much of the research on wheatgrass has been conducted in Japan, American scientists have also hailed this green food for its many benefits. One important study performed by Dr. Arthur Robinson at the Oregon Institute of Science and Medicine found that wheatgrass and other "live foods" decreased the incidence and severity of cancer lesions in mice by about 75 percent. In a 1978 study, Dr. Chiu-Nan Lai of the University of Texas reported in Nutrition and Cancer that wheatgrass had an antimutagenic effect and that it also showed antineoplastic ability.

Wheatgrass has also been shown to have beneficial external effects with topical application, being used successfully to treat such disorders as skin ulcers, impetigo, and itching.

TRADITIONAL AND OTHER THERAPEUTIC USES

- cleanses blood and internal organs
- stimulates metabolism
- aids in weight loss
- possibly helps resist cancer
- improves skin conditions (topical)
- supplies important vitamins and other nutrients

YOHIMBE

ORIGIN
Africa

PART OF PLANT USED
Bark

DESCRIPTION
Yohimbe is a tree that grows throughout the African nations of Cameroon, Gabon and Zaire. For centuries, natives from these areas have ingested both the crude bark and purified compound as a tonic to enhance sexual prowess and as an aphrodisiac. The bark has been smoked as a hallucinogen and has been used in traditional medicine to treat angina and hypertension. The herb is a sensual stimulant for both men and women. Today, doctors prescribe an extract from the tree to treat organic impotence.

Yohimbe has energizing effects that stem from its ability to increase blood flow to the genitals, both male and female. It is thought to stimulate the pelvic nerve ganglia and thus is helpful for men with erection problems. In fact, a prescription drug, yohimbine hydrochloride, is the only FDA approved drug for impotence. Effects can include increased libido, sensation, and stamina. Women have also reported similar effects and general pleasant sensations.

Yohimbe bark contains about 6% yohimbine. This constituent is an indole alkaloid that is classified as an alpha-2-adrenergic blocking agent. The herb is a general nervous system stimulant and can cause changes in blood pressure by dilating blood vessels. It can increase the heart rate, raise body temperature and even increase blood pressure. At higher doses, yohimbe has a mild psychotropic effect.

Yohimbe bark stimulates chemical reactions in the body that may aid in psychogenic cases of impotence, due to fatigue, tension and stress. Clinical studies have shown the herb to be effective in restoring potency in diabetic and heart patients who suffer from impotence. Yohimbe expands the blood vessels not only to the genitals (similar to the prescription drug Viagra), but also to the skin and even fat cells. As an alpha-2-adrenergic blocker, yohimbe reduces the effect of hormones that cause constriction of blood vessels, which typically increases as we age. It increases the body's production of norepinephrine, which is essential for proper erectile function. Yohimbe may boost the adrenaline (epinephrine) supply to nerve endings as well, which can enhance sensual stimulation. Yohimbe also inhibits serotonin. When serotonin levels increase, blood pressure, exhaustion, depression and nervousness also increase which inhibit sexual performance.

Yohimbe is also a short term MAO (monoamine oxidase) inhibitor and should be used with caution, especially if you have high blood pressure. Being an MAO inhibitor, yohimbe should not be taken with any food or drink containing tyramines (cheese, chocolate, beer and nuts).

Yohimbe has been recommended in sports medicine for male athletes, especially body builders, for its supposed effect of increasing blood levels of the male hormone testosterone, which can cause an anabolic or muscle building effect.

TRADITIONAL AND OTHER THERAPEUTIC USES
- treats impotence
- aphrodisiac
- seems to increase testosterone

TOXICITY, CAUTIONS AND CONTRAINDICATIONS
Anyone with a heart condition, kidney disease, hypertension, glaucoma or history of gastric or duodenal ulcers should avoid this herb. As mentioned above, yohimbe should not be taken with any food or drink containing tyramines (e.g, cheese, chocolate, beer and nuts).

WILD YAM
(Dioscorea villosa L.)

ORIGIN
Mexico, India, China, Peru and Africa

PART OF PLANT USED
Root

DESCRIPTION
Wild yam has a long history of use as both a food and a medicine. Its key constituents are diosgenin, saponins, tannins, catechins, indoles, glucosides, and oligopolysaccharides. Diosgenin, a steroidal glycoside, is partially converted in the intestines to the hormones DHEA, 6-ketodiosgenin and 9-ketodiosgenin. DHEA is the most abundant adrenal steroid hormone in the body and is also produced in the ovaries prior to menopause. It is a precursor for estrogen, testosterone, and other hormones, as well as having functions of its own. Its production in the body is known to decrease steadily with age, especially in women with the onset of menopause. In fact, many degenerative conditions are associated with lower than normal levels of DHEA. These conditions include cardiovascular disease, high cholesterol, diabetes, obesity, cancer, Alzheimer's disease and other memory disturbances, immune system disorders including HIV, and chronic fatigue syndrome.

Increased availability of DHEA may either directly modulate the action of corticosteroids, or simply reduce the indirect side effects caused by a reduction in DHEA levels that accompany the use of corticosteroids. This may result in a reduction in the incidence and severity of osteoporosis brought on by the use of corticosteroids.

TRADITIONAL AND OTHER THERAPEUTIC USES

- dysmenorrhea, menopausal symptoms, and ovarian/uterine pain
- mild diaphoretic
- anti-inflammatory and anti-rheumatic
- spasmolytic, sometimes helpful with muscular rheumatism and cramps
- cholagogue sometimes helpful in cholecystitis
- treats intestinal colic, diverticulitis, , and intermittent claudication

TOXICITY, CAUTIONS AND CONTRAINDICATIONS

Not for use by pregnant women. Wild yam root is non-toxic, but is contraindicated for known or suspected prostate cancer. Although it does not contain anabolic steroids, it is advisable for sports competitors to check whether their sport tests for DHEA, 6-ketodiosgenin or 9-ketodiosgenin, or whether those compounds might cause a false positive result under the drug-testing regimen used.

WILLOW BARK
(Salix alba)

ORIGIN
Worldwide; S. alba (white willow), native to Eurasia and Africa, now grows wild in North America

PART OF PLANT USED
Bark

DESCRIPTION
The bark of the common willow tree has been used since antiquity for its pain-relieving and fever-reducing properties. In the early 19th century, a French chemist extracted its principal active ingredient and named it "salicin." At the end of the century, Felix Hofmann, a chemist at the Bayer pharmaceutical company in Germany, developed the world's most used medicine, aspirin, also known as acetylsalicylic acid. Recently, pain sufferers are returning to the natural source to avoid the potentially dangerous side effects of aspirin.

Salicin is a bitter phenolic glycoside, a monoglycoside of salycilic acid. Salicylic acid is a weak anti-inflammatory agent, converted by the liver into acetylsalicylic acid. This natural conversion process in the body avoids the gastrointestinal upset associated with direct ingestion of synthetic aspirin. The salicylates inhibit the activity of the cyclo-oxygenase enzyme, thus inhibiting the production of prostaglandins and other inflammatory molecules.

In topical application, extracts and infusions of willow bark have long been used to clean the scalp and skin, and to treat dandruff, corns, and growths. Like its synthesized descendant, aspirin, it is useful against warts. The astringency of the glycosides also makes willow bark useful as an antiseptic.

TRADITIONAL AND OTHER THERAPEUTIC USES

- temporary pain relief in headache, menstrual pain, toothache, arthritis, gout, and sore muscles
- treats fevers
- treats inflammatory and rheumatic pain
- beneficial for connective tissue disorders
- antiseptic for urinary tract infections and intestinal worms and parasites
- useful as an astringent for dysentery and diarrhea

TOXICITY, CAUTIONS AND CONTRAINDICATIONS

None known. Use by children should be avoided. Individuals allergic to salicylates should avoid willow bark.

Index

C

F

G

H

K

L

M

SPECIAL DEDICATION TO
LINUS PAULING,
NOBEL LAUREATE

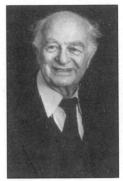

Many times, I met Linus Pauling in between 1984 and 1994 in different conventions and personal meetings as a Publisher of Health World magazine. Dr. Pauling told me, many things in modern medicine and surgery have derived from Charak Samhita and Sushruta Samhita of Ayurvedic medicine in India, which is the oldest system of medical science. Doctors and surgeons were quite well trained 10,000 years back in ancient India. I was quite surprise to know what he knew about Ayurvedic Medical Science. He told me, Ayurvedic is the life science of human being.

I really loved him so much, the way he always talked to me about his Vitamin C theory. Even he would listen to me a lot about Ayurvedic Medicine too.. The late Linus Pauling was the only in the world to have won two times unshared Nobel Prizes. In 1954, for Chemistry and 1962, for peace. Two Nobel Prizes by one man in one life time! Linus Pauling was globally admired and controversial globally..

Dr.Pauling candidly spoke his mind about peace to presidents, heads of state and all others alike. He hated war and found it unacceptable. He shared his devotion to pacifism with his friend Albert Einstein, in 1958, he presented a petition, which was signed by 11,000 scientists, warning the public about the biological danger of radioactive fallout from nuclear weapons testing

World Peace was Pauling's passion, but he was equally as dedicated to chemistry as it helps humanity. His 1954 Nobel Prize was awarded for his work on genetic influences in relation to the atomic structure of proteins in hemoglobin. He discovered that sickle cell anemia is caused by genetic defect. Professor Linus Pauling was considered the Champion of Vitamin C and its curative powers in immune system.

He continued his other scientific work at the Linus Pauling Institute of Science and Medicine in Palo Alto, California. There, he and 35 other researchers researched the basic mechanisms of disease, including the way to decipher human genes.

He used to take 10,000mg (10 grams) of Vitamin C everyday.

I learned a lot from this great man, Dr. Pauling and I pray for his eternal soul.

Linus Pauling died in 1994 at the age of 93.